Acknowledgements

Several associates worked on this story and added to its creation namely,
Jesica Medellin and Linda McLean, editors, Lori Taylor, illustrator, and Streetlight Graphics.

This book is dedicated to my totally Irish grandmother, Alice Cecelia (Maher) Palmer,
The Maher Clan, and all who believe in "the wee folk".

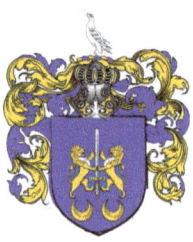

Fairies and the Global Tree to the Rescue:
A Tale of the Fairy Flu
Copyright © 2020 by Carol Trembath

Paperback ISBN: 978-0-9907446-9-6
Hardcover ISBN: 978-1-7360457-0-1
Ebooks ISBN: 978-1-7360457-1-8

Illustrations by Lori Taylor

Lakeside Publishing MI

Printed in the United States of America

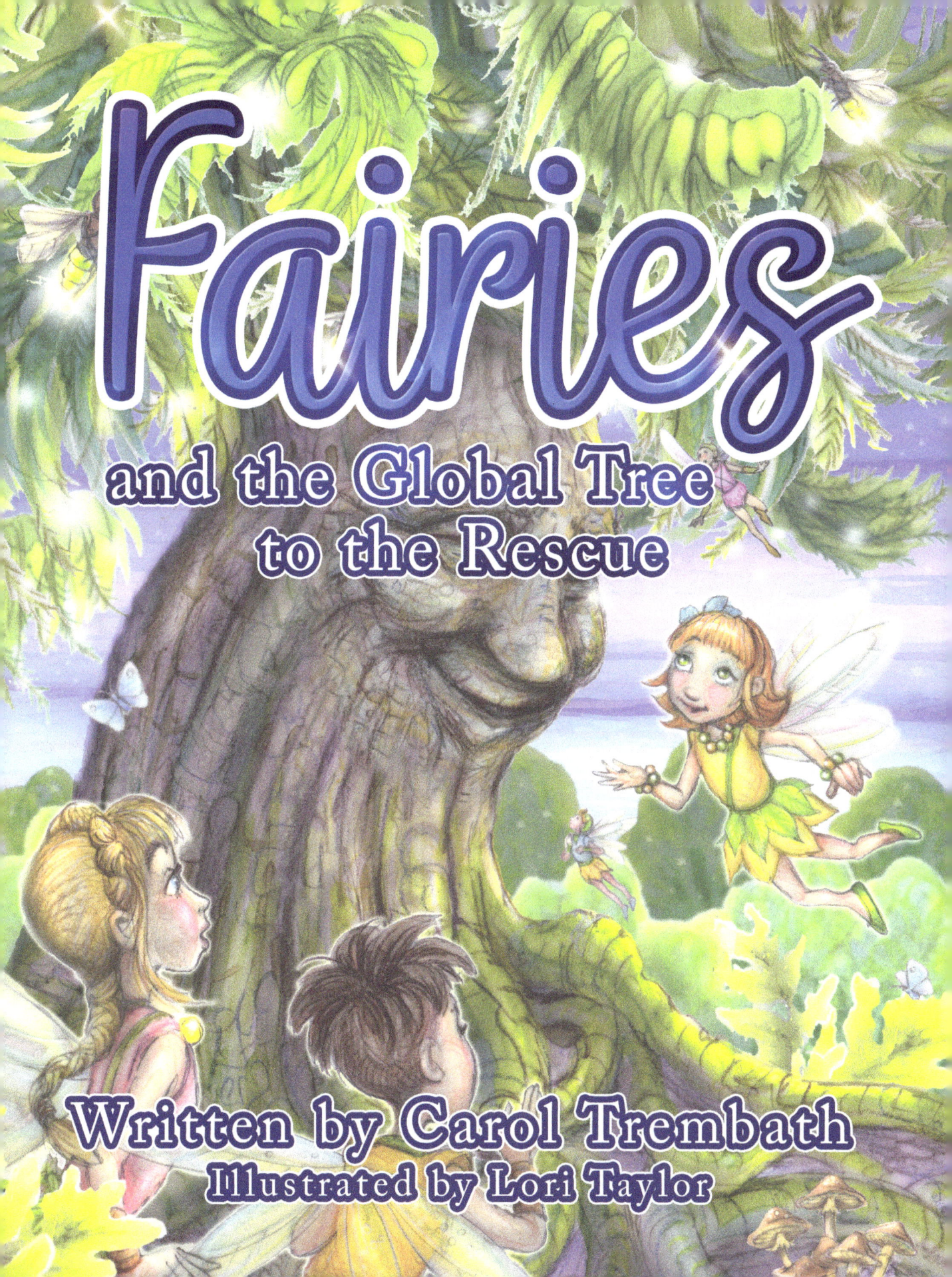

Fairies

and the Global Tree
to the Rescue

Written by Carol Trembath
Illustrated by Lori Taylor

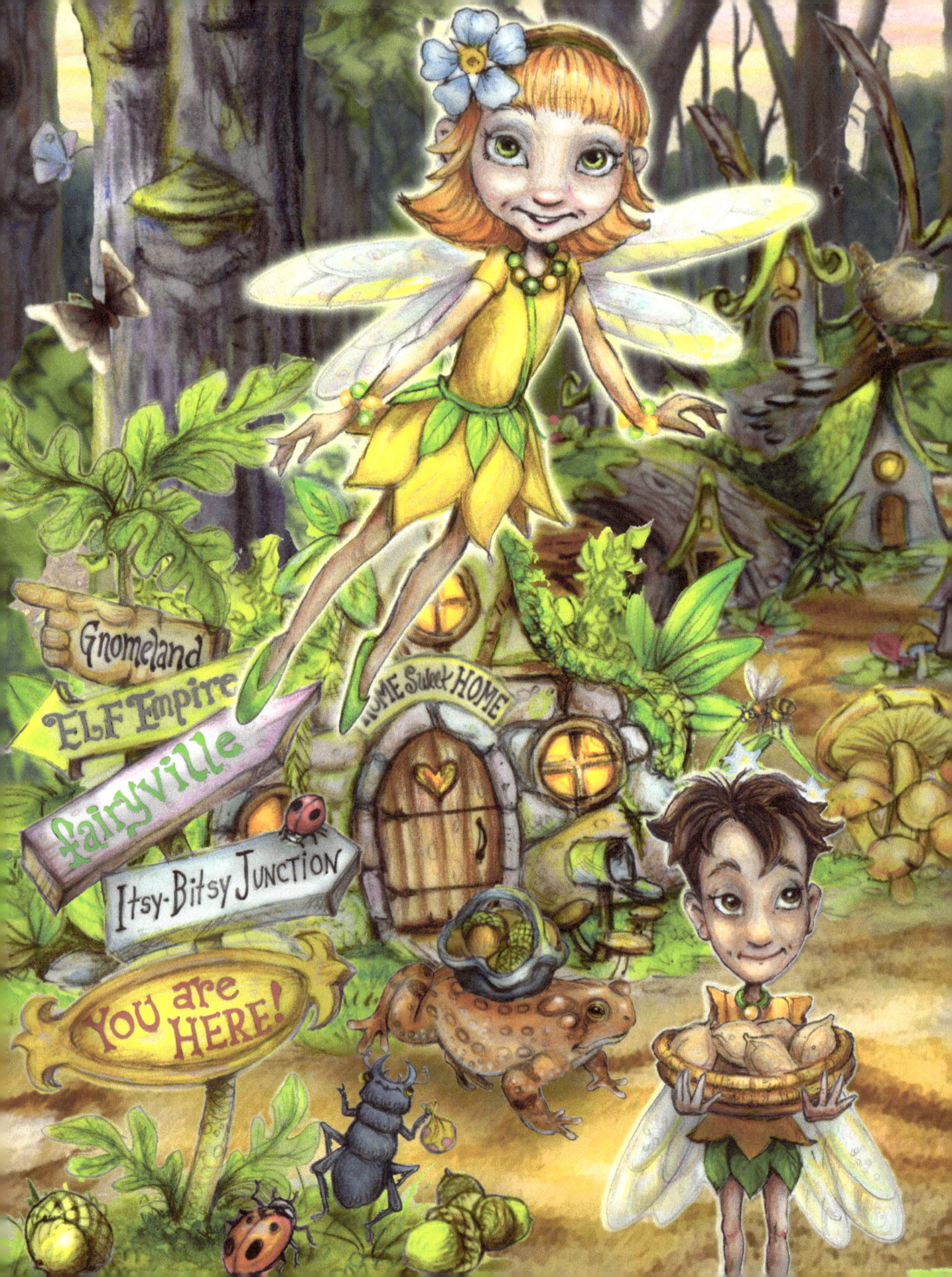

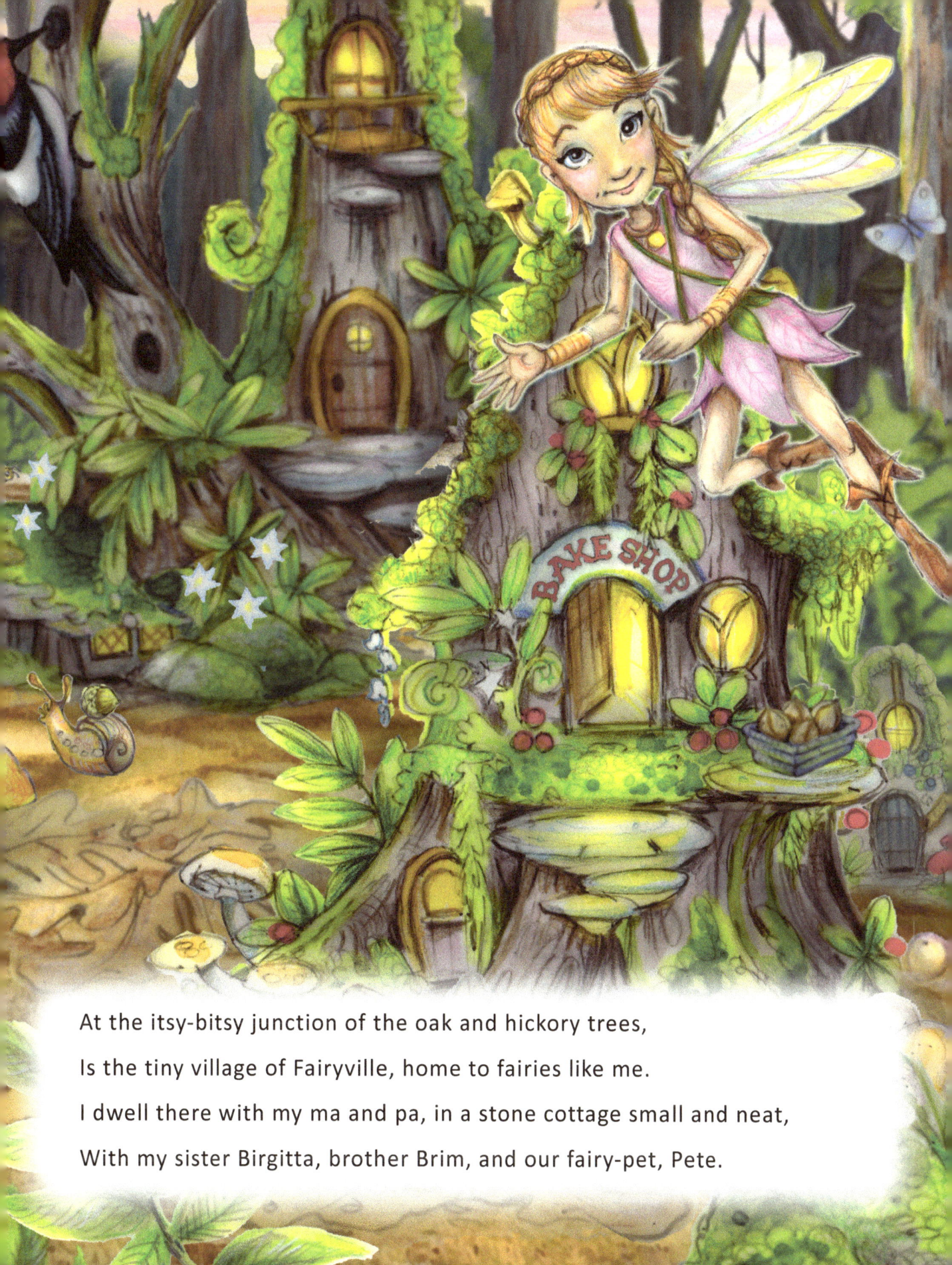

At the itsy-bitsy junction of the oak and hickory trees,

Is the tiny village of Fairyville, home to fairies like me.

I dwell there with my ma and pa, in a stone cottage small and neat,

With my sister Birgitta, brother Brim, and our fairy-pet, Pete.

Each day begins with a visit to Finnegan at the bakeshop.

He says, "Hello, Tinsley, here is a goody with sprinkles on top."

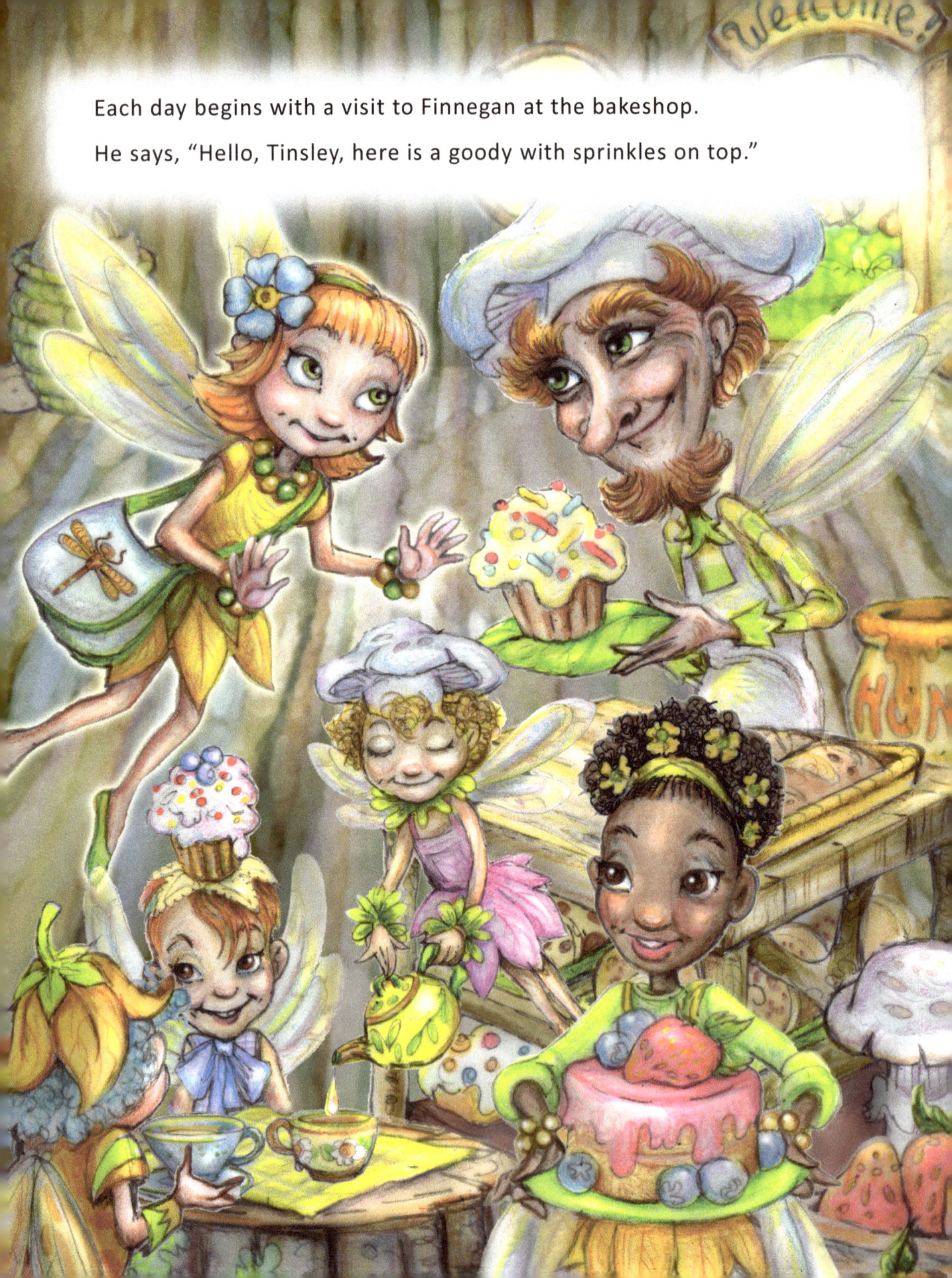

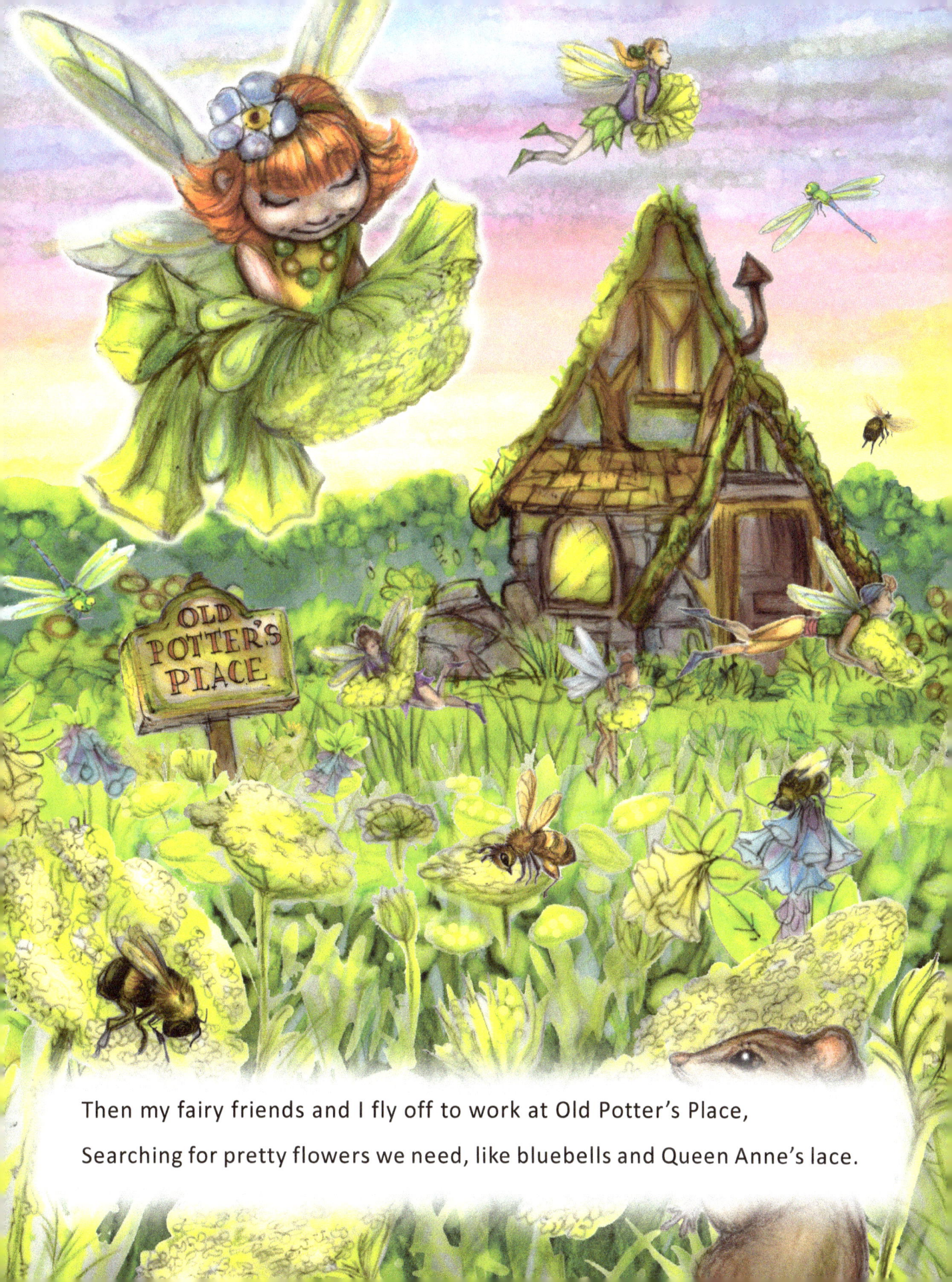

Then my fairy friends and I fly off to work at Old Potter's Place,

Searching for pretty flowers we need, like bluebells and Queen Anne's lace.

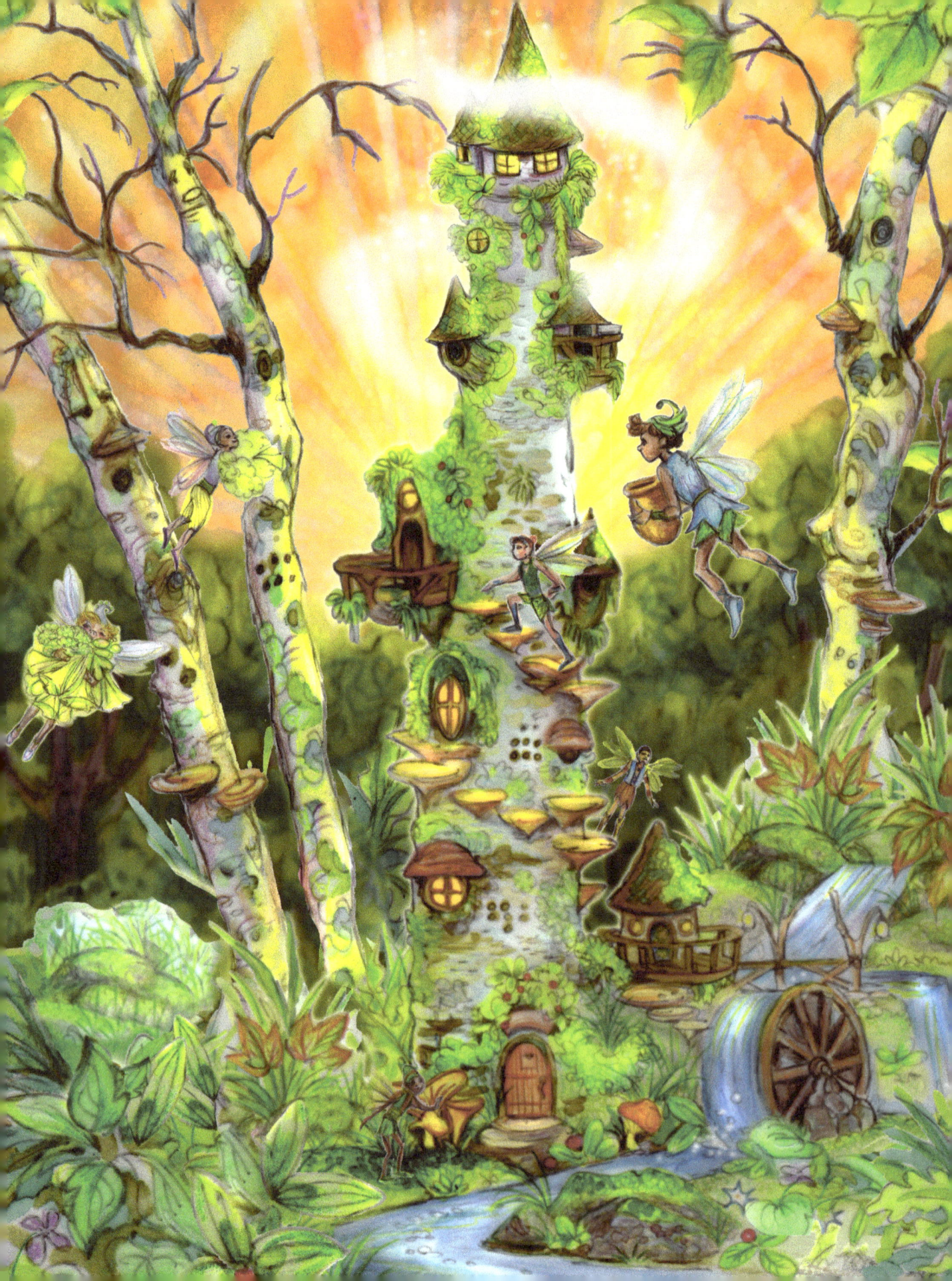

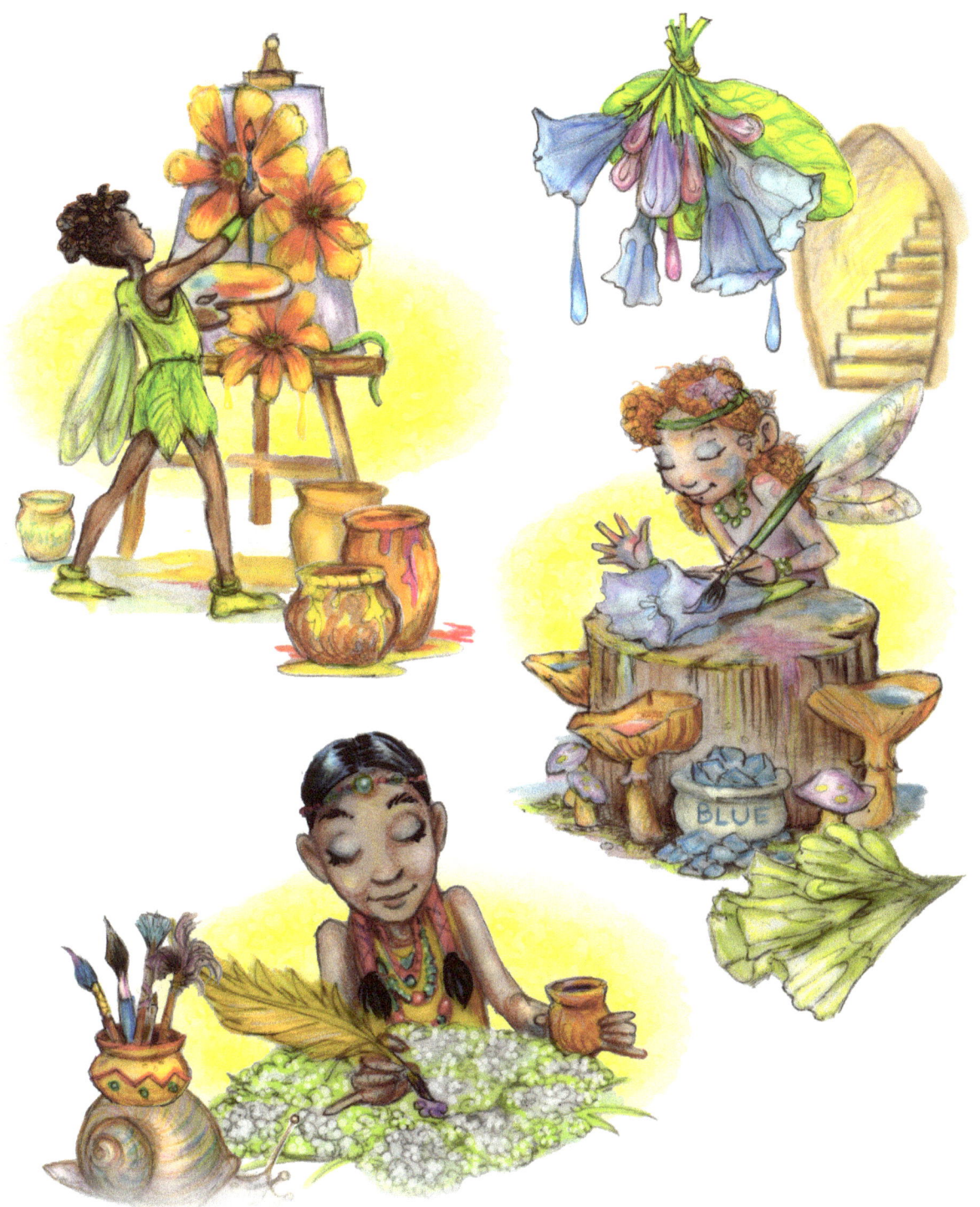

We take our bouquets to Fairy Tower and climb the hidden stair,

To deliver them to the artists where they're painted with great care.

My friends and I are curious about the top of the tower,

The place they make the fairy dust that gives us our flying power.

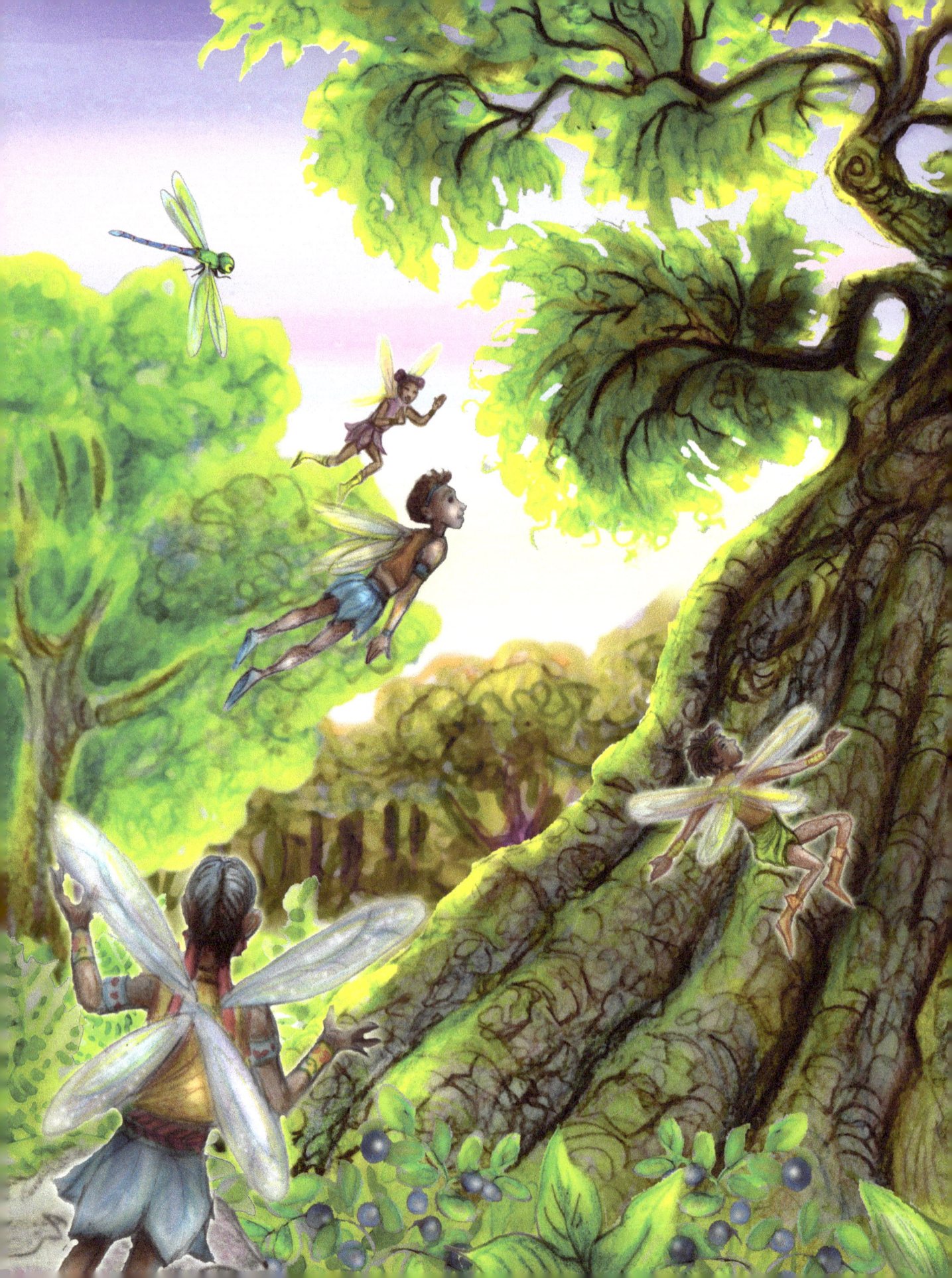

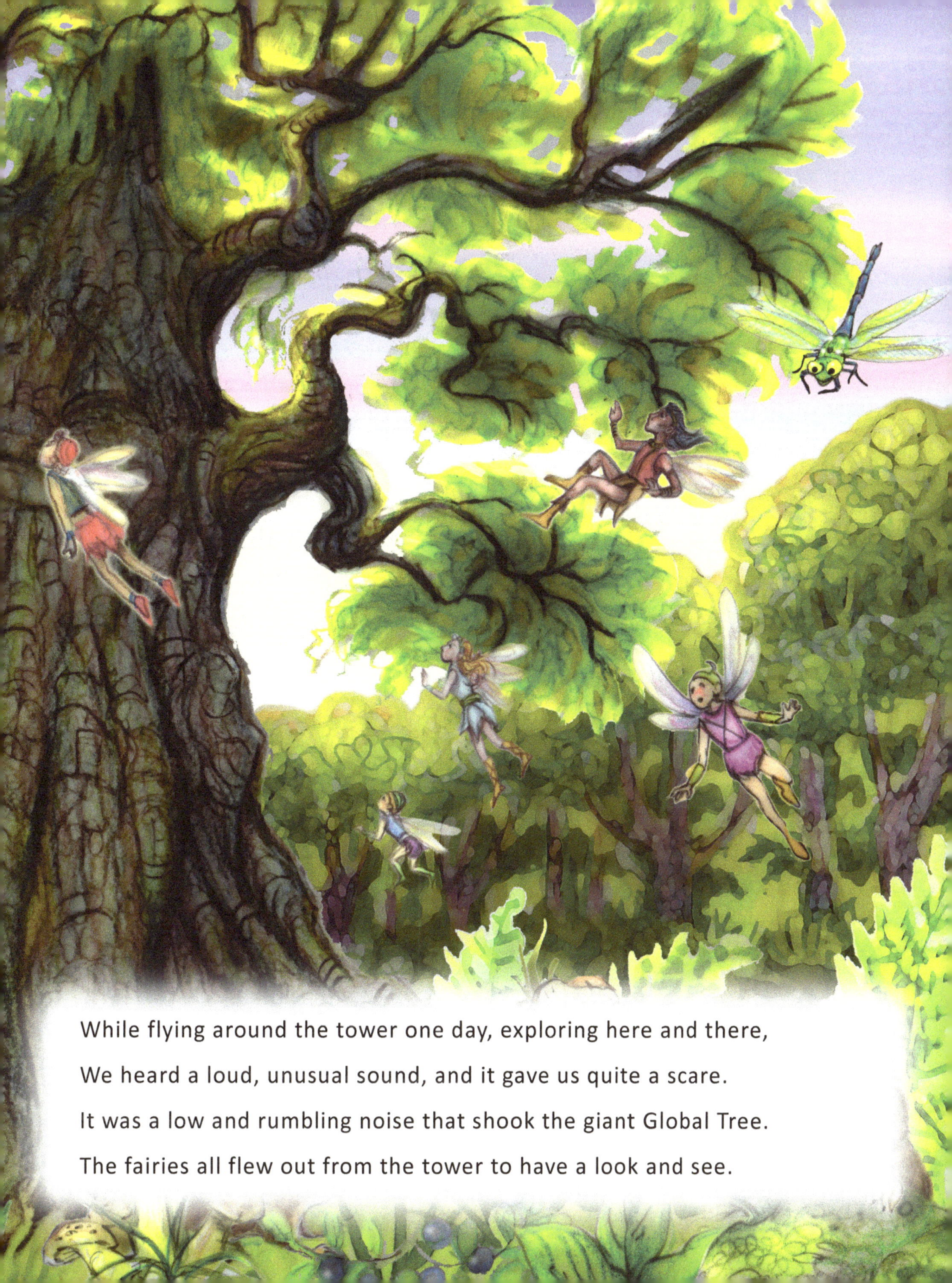

While flying around the tower one day, exploring here and there,

We heard a loud, unusual sound, and it gave us quite a scare.

It was a low and rumbling noise that shook the giant Global Tree.

The fairies all flew out from the tower to have a look and see.

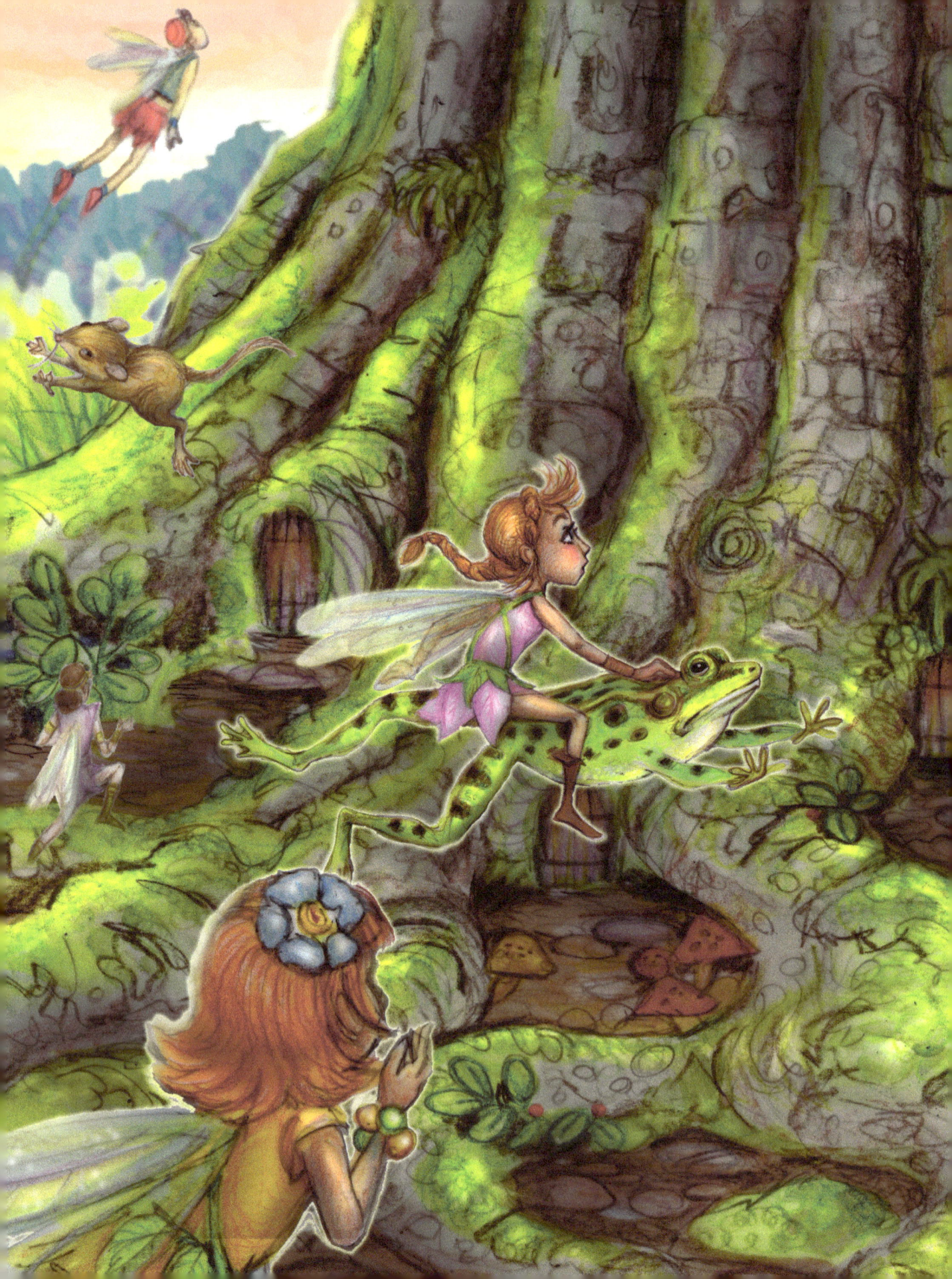

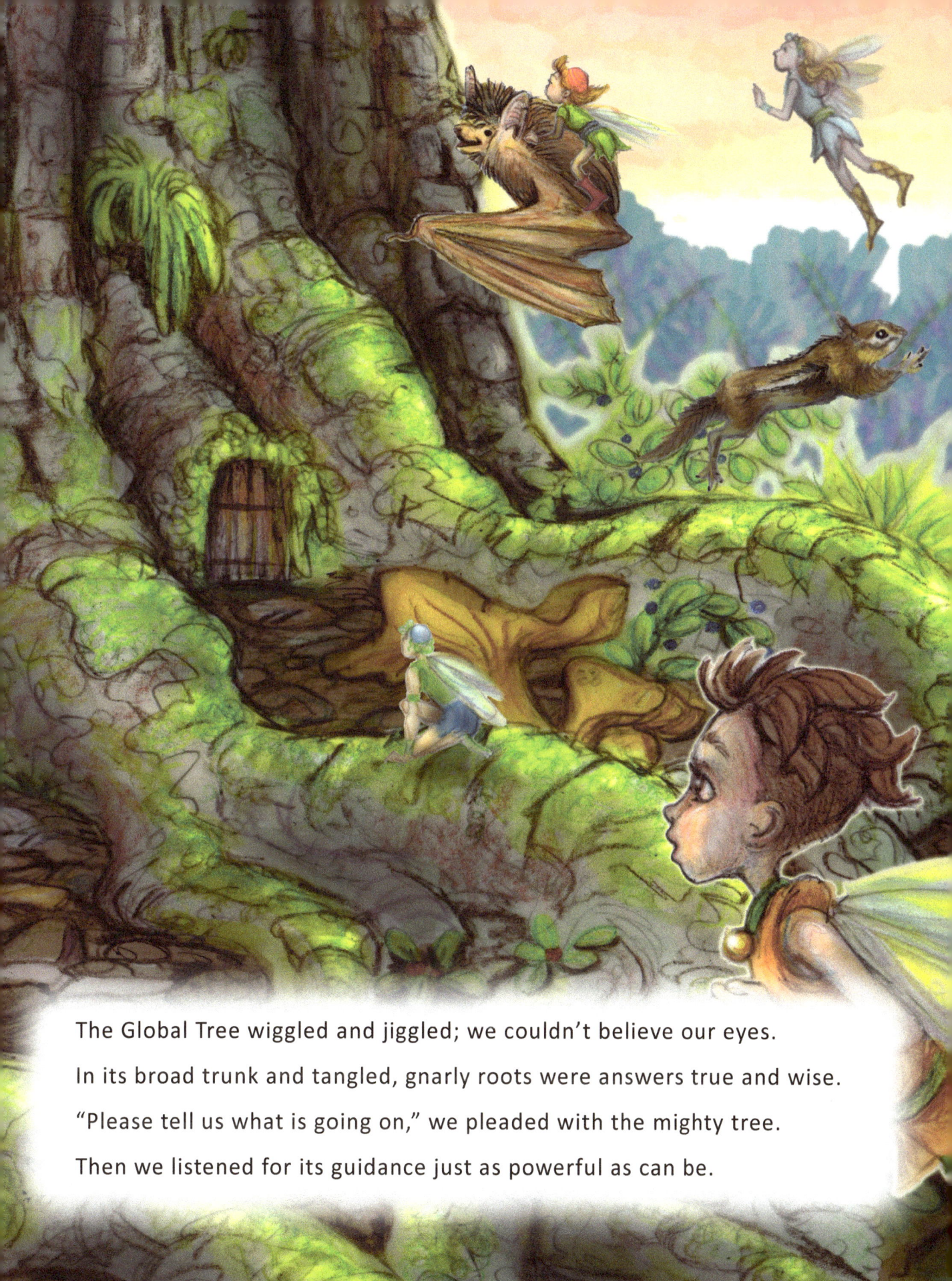

The Global Tree wiggled and jiggled; we couldn't believe our eyes.

In its broad trunk and tangled, gnarly roots were answers true and wise.

"Please tell us what is going on," we pleaded with the mighty tree.

Then we listened for its guidance just as powerful as can be.

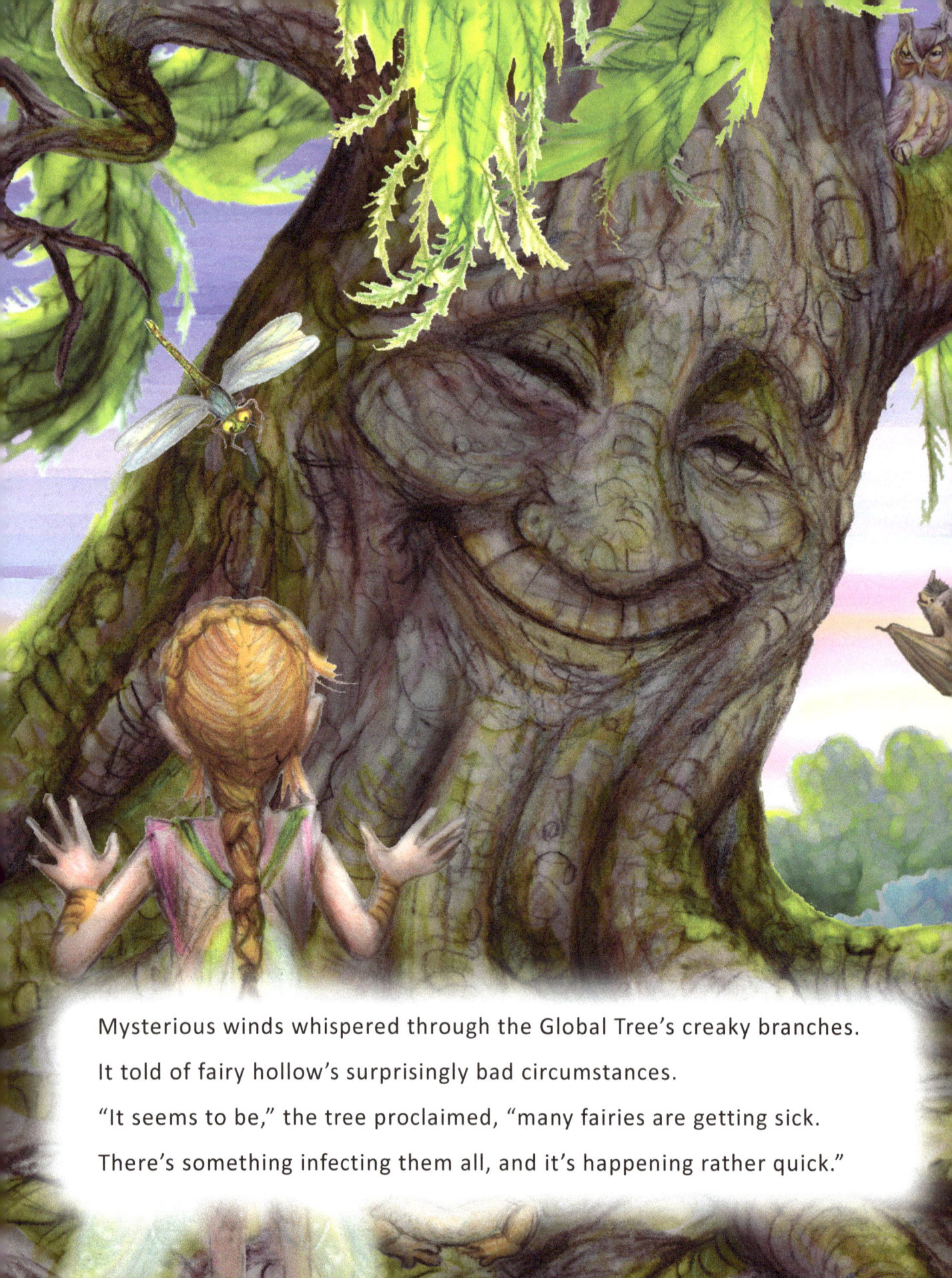

Mysterious winds whispered through the Global Tree's creaky branches.

It told of fairy hollow's surprisingly bad circumstances.

"It seems to be," the tree proclaimed, "many fairies are getting sick.

There's something infecting them all, and it's happening rather quick."

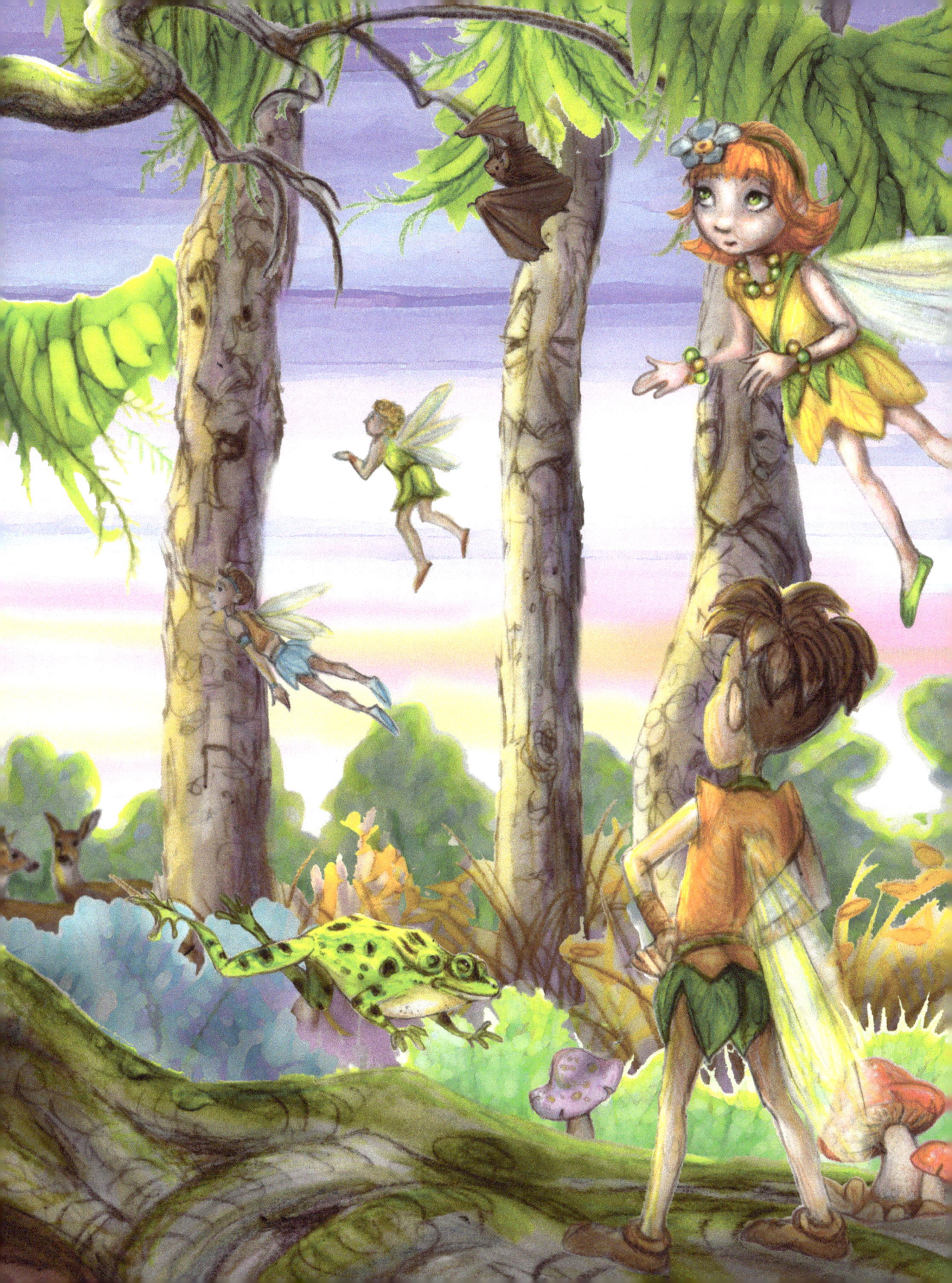

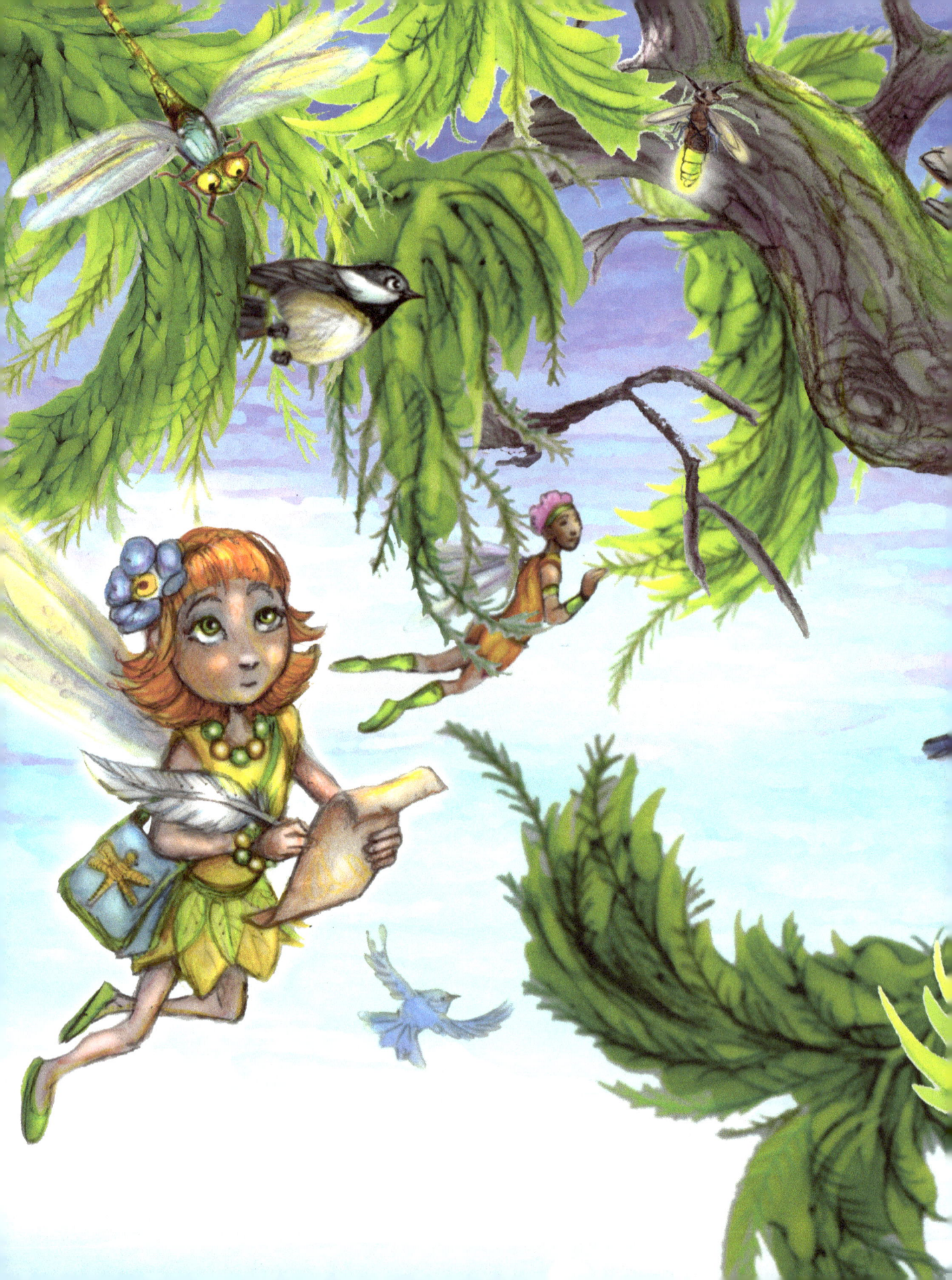

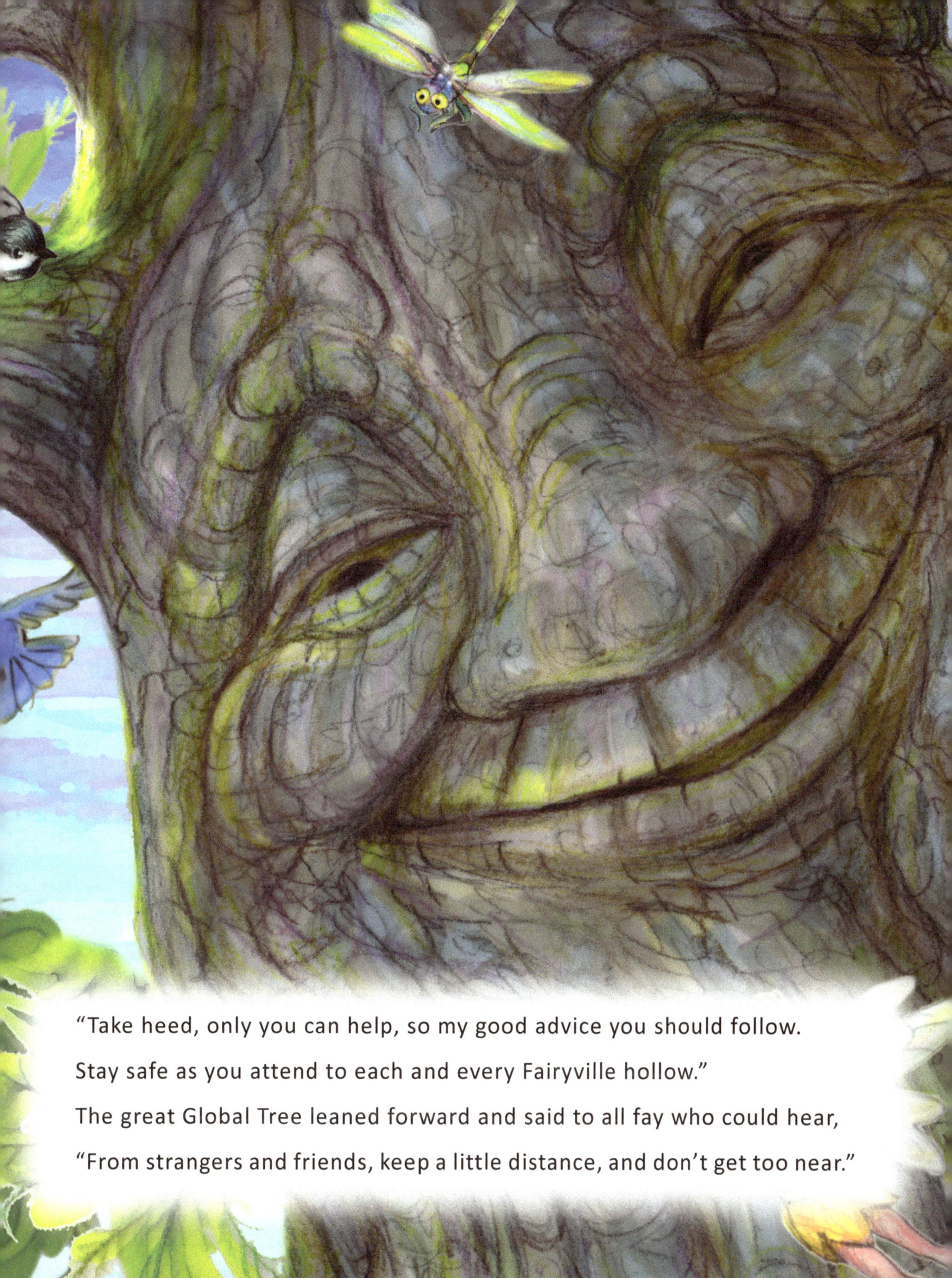

"Take heed, only you can help, so my good advice you should follow.

Stay safe as you attend to each and every Fairyville hollow."

The great Global Tree leaned forward and said to all fay who could hear,

"From strangers and friends, keep a little distance, and don't get too near."

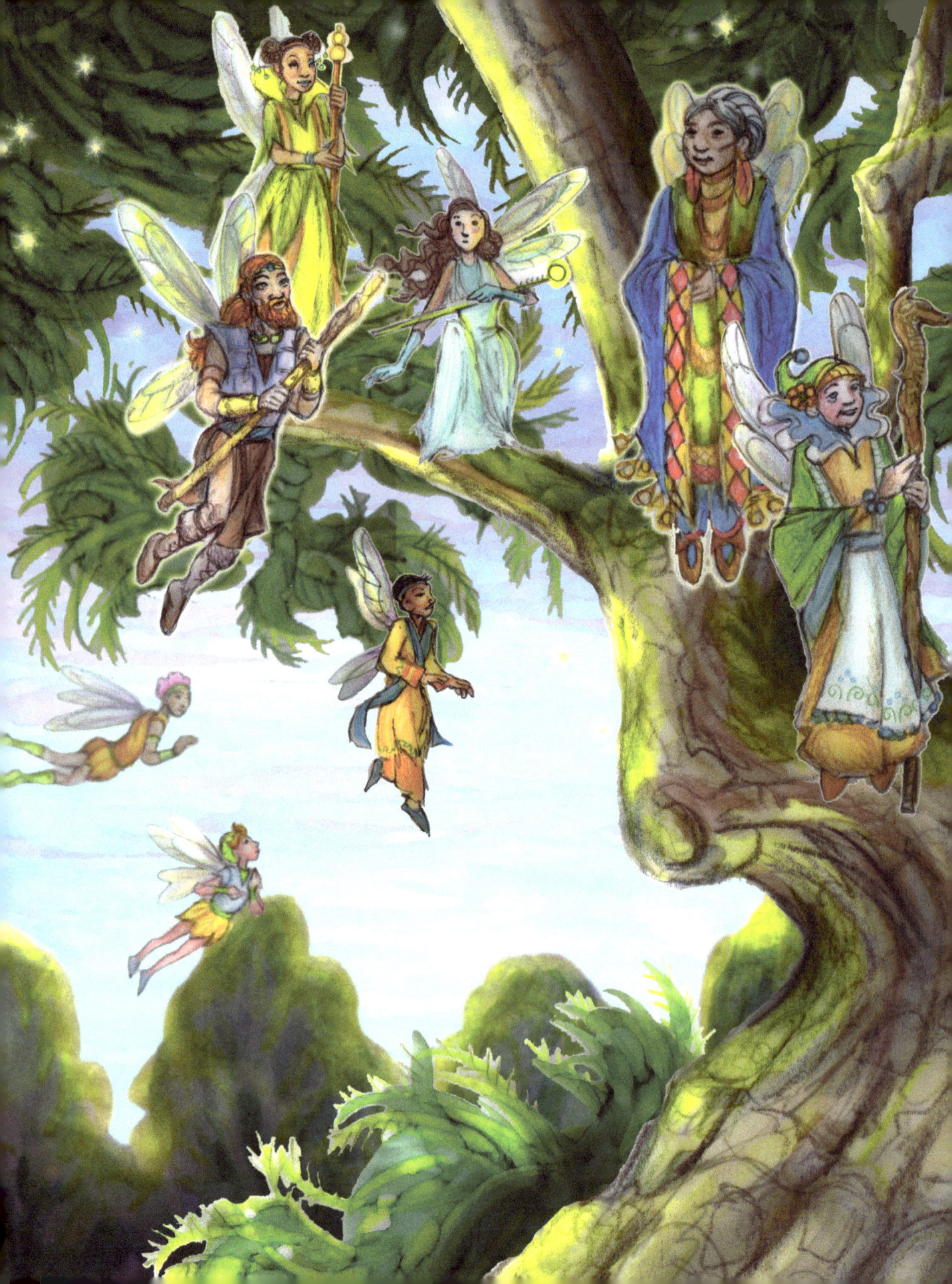

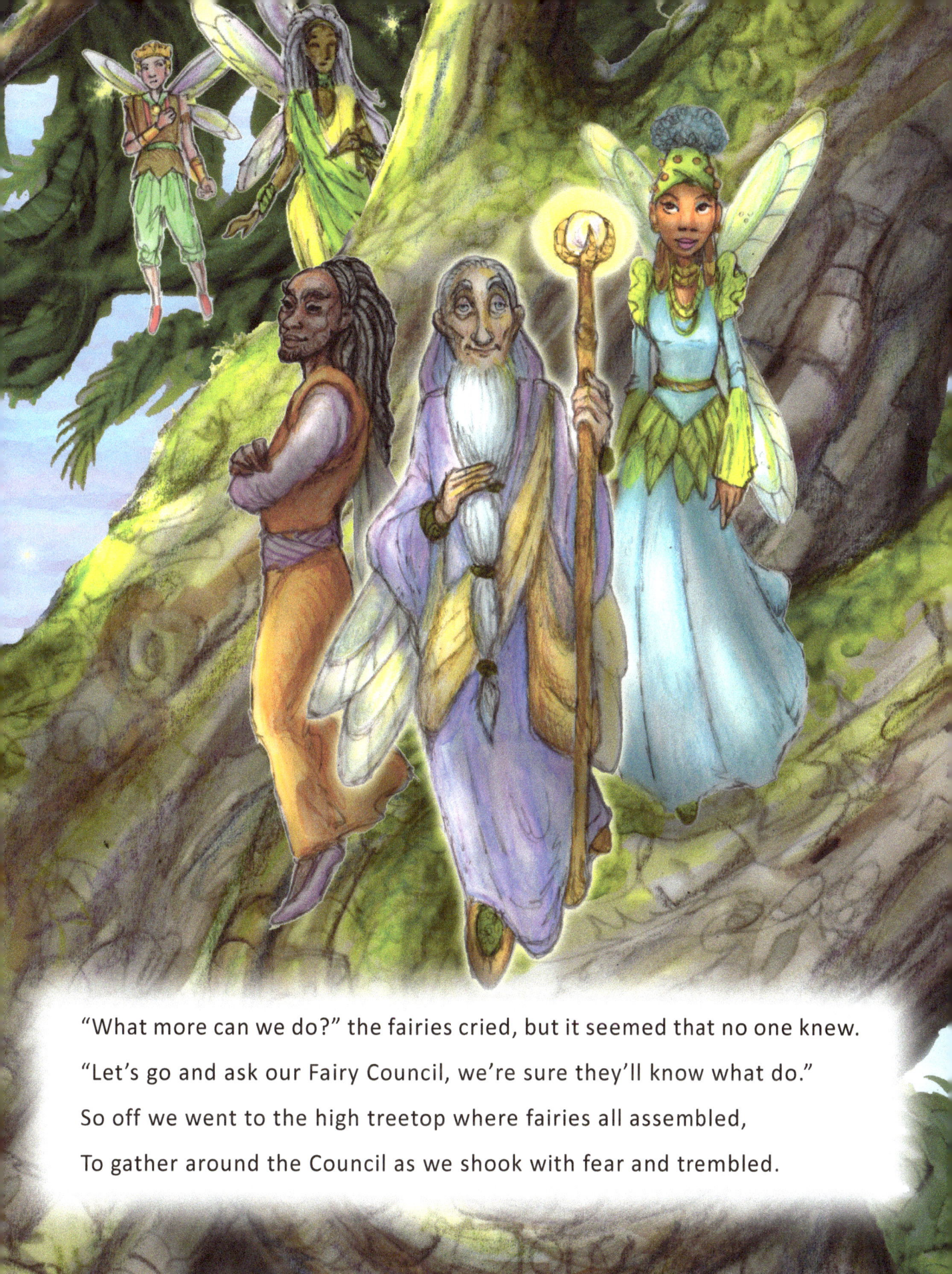

"What more can we do?" the fairies cried, but it seemed that no one knew.

"Let's go and ask our Fairy Council, we're sure they'll know what do."

So off we went to the high treetop where fairies all assembled,

To gather around the Council as we shook with fear and trembled.

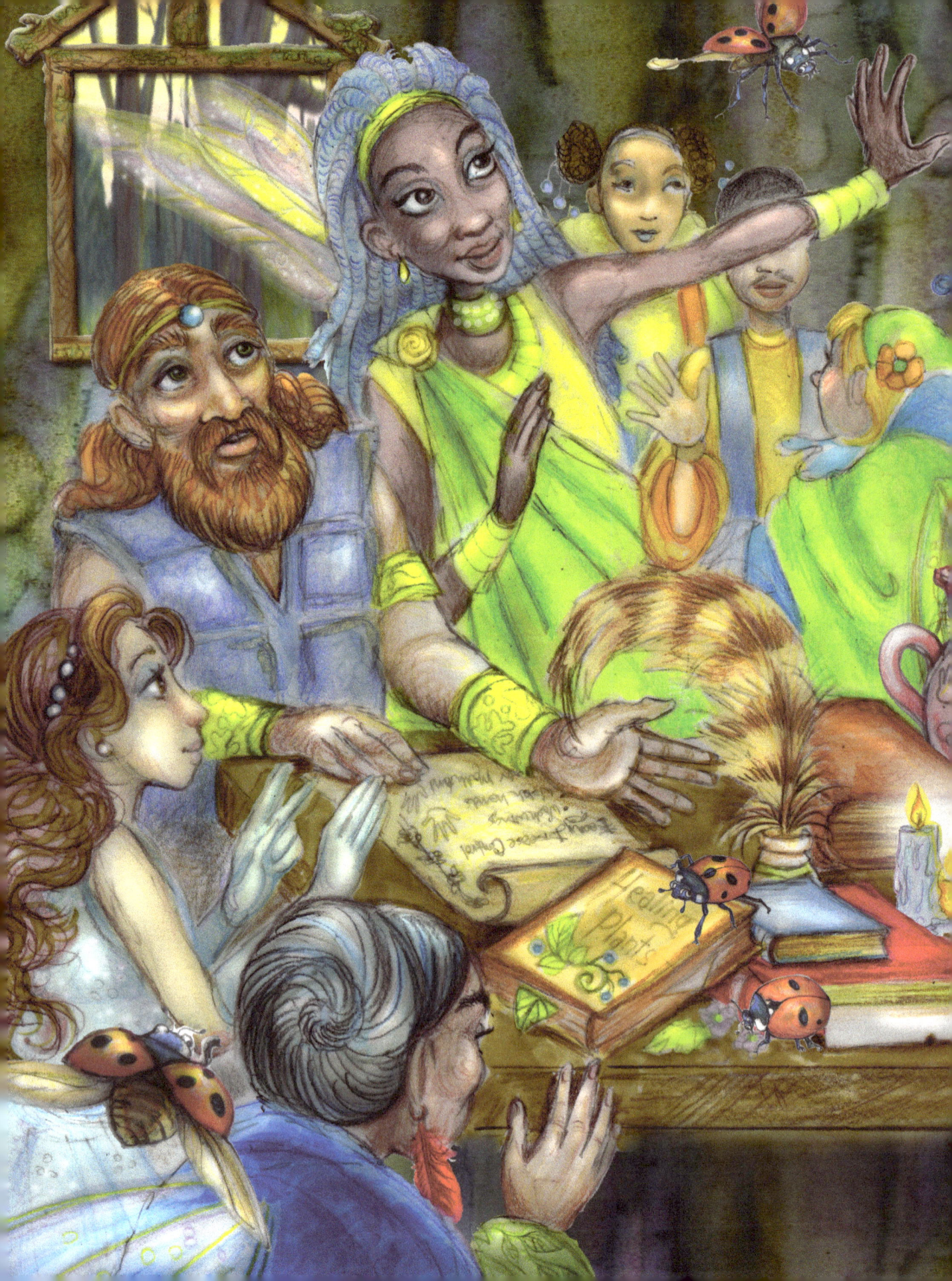

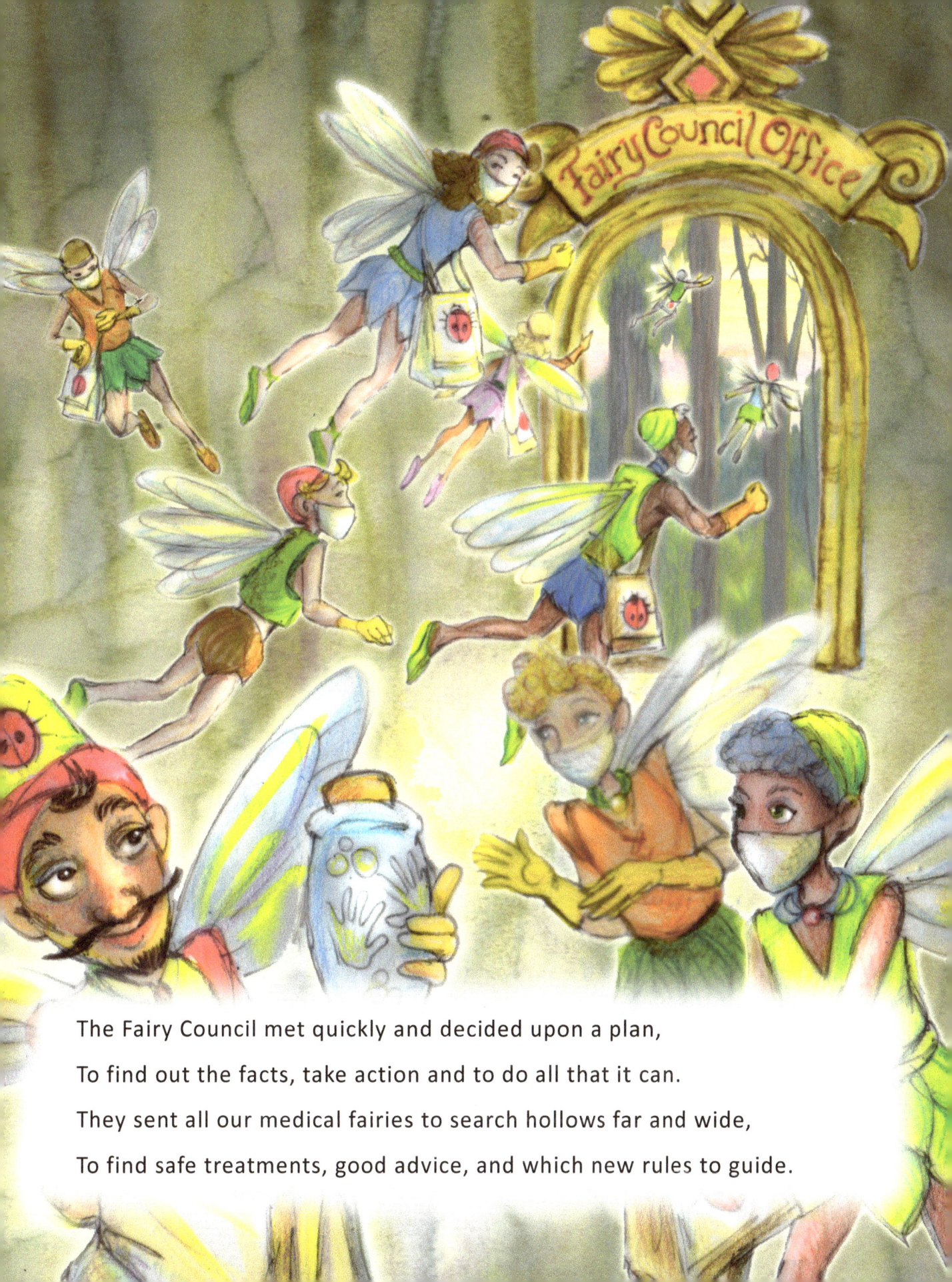

The Fairy Council met quickly and decided upon a plan,

To find out the facts, take action and to do all that it can.

They sent all our medical fairies to search hollows far and wide,

To find safe treatments, good advice, and which new rules to guide.

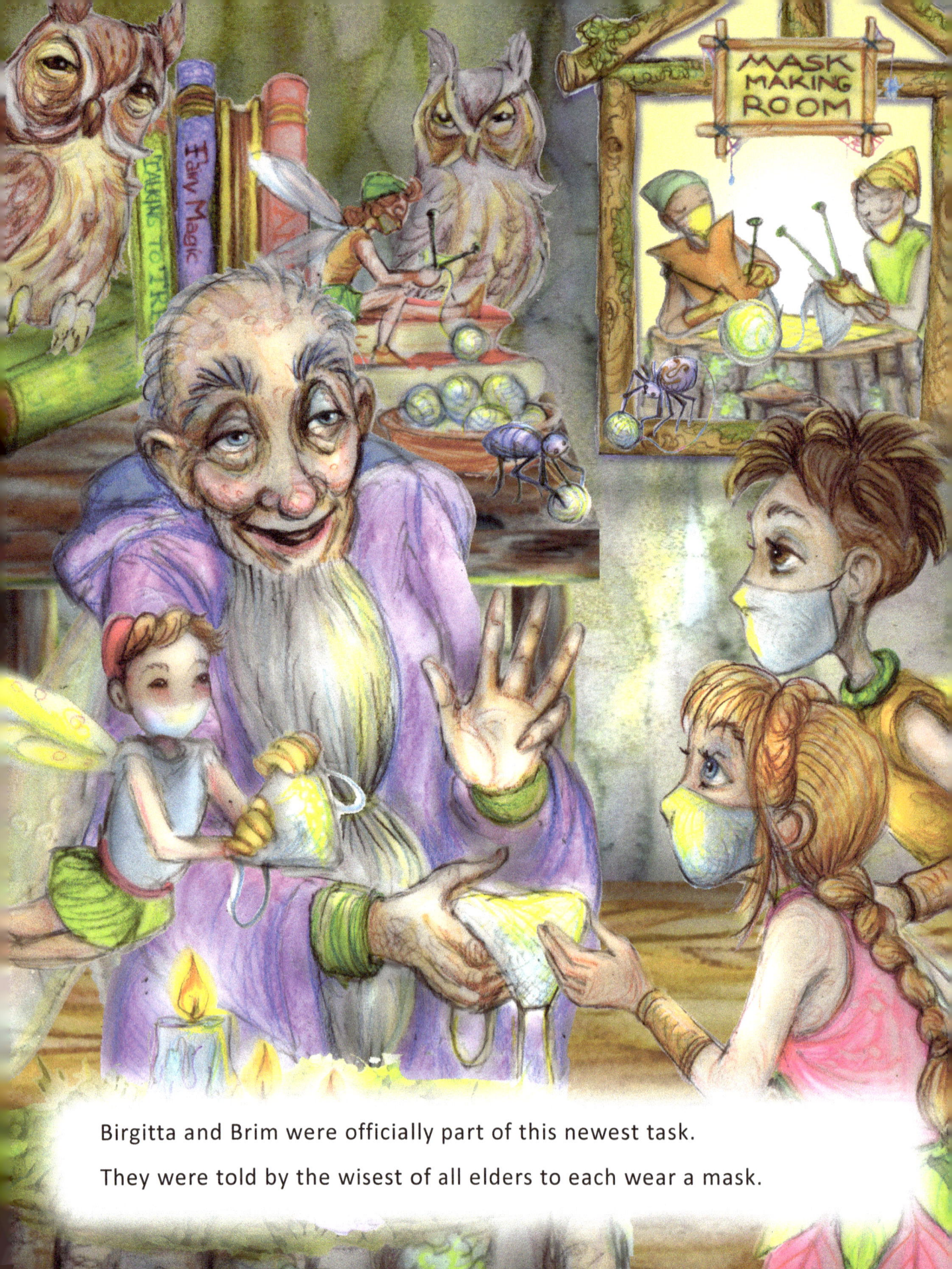

Birgitta and Brim were officially part of this newest task.

They were told by the wisest of all elders to each wear a mask.

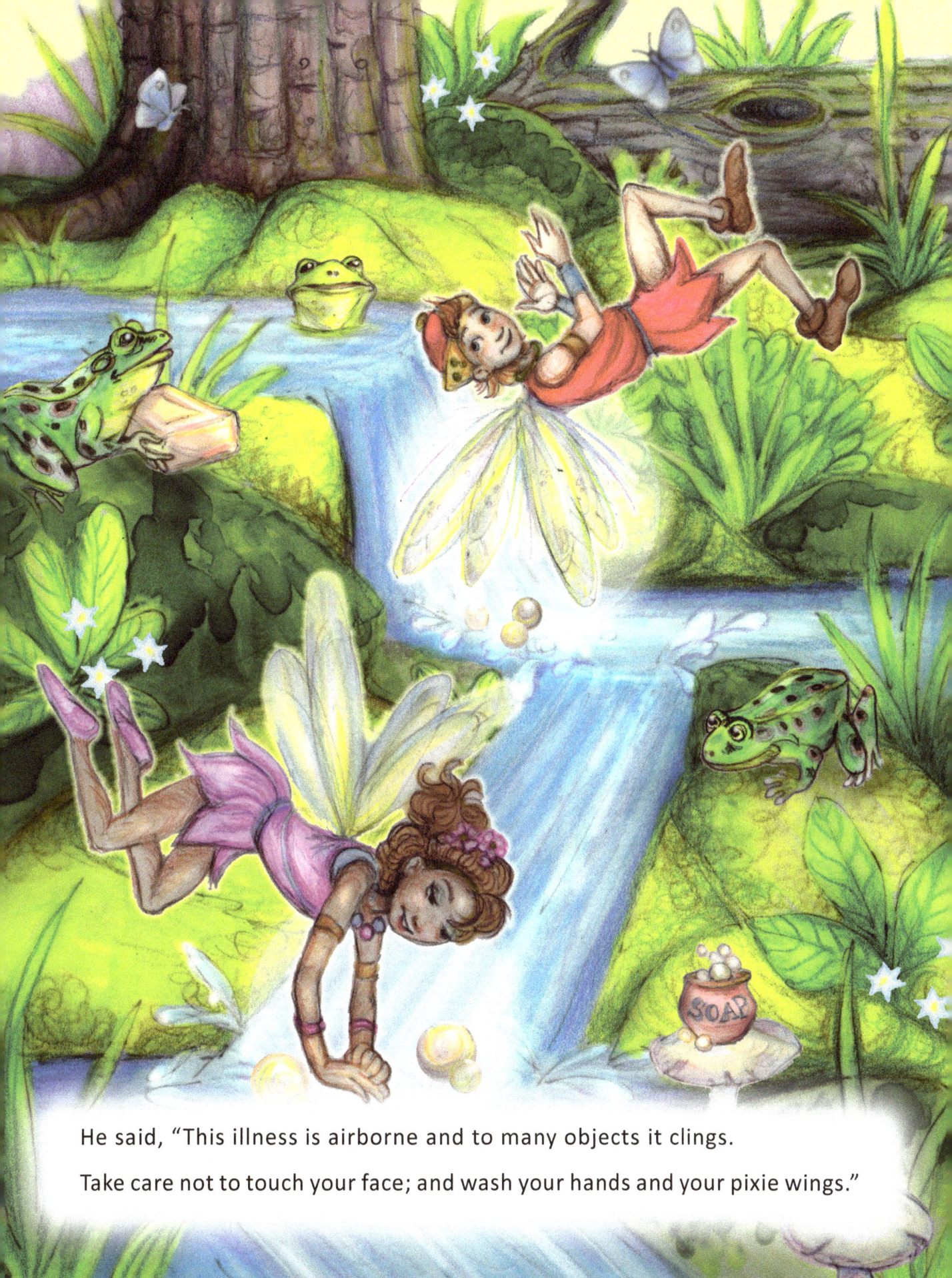

He said, "This illness is airborne and to many objects it clings.

Take care not to touch your face; and wash your hands and your pixie wings."

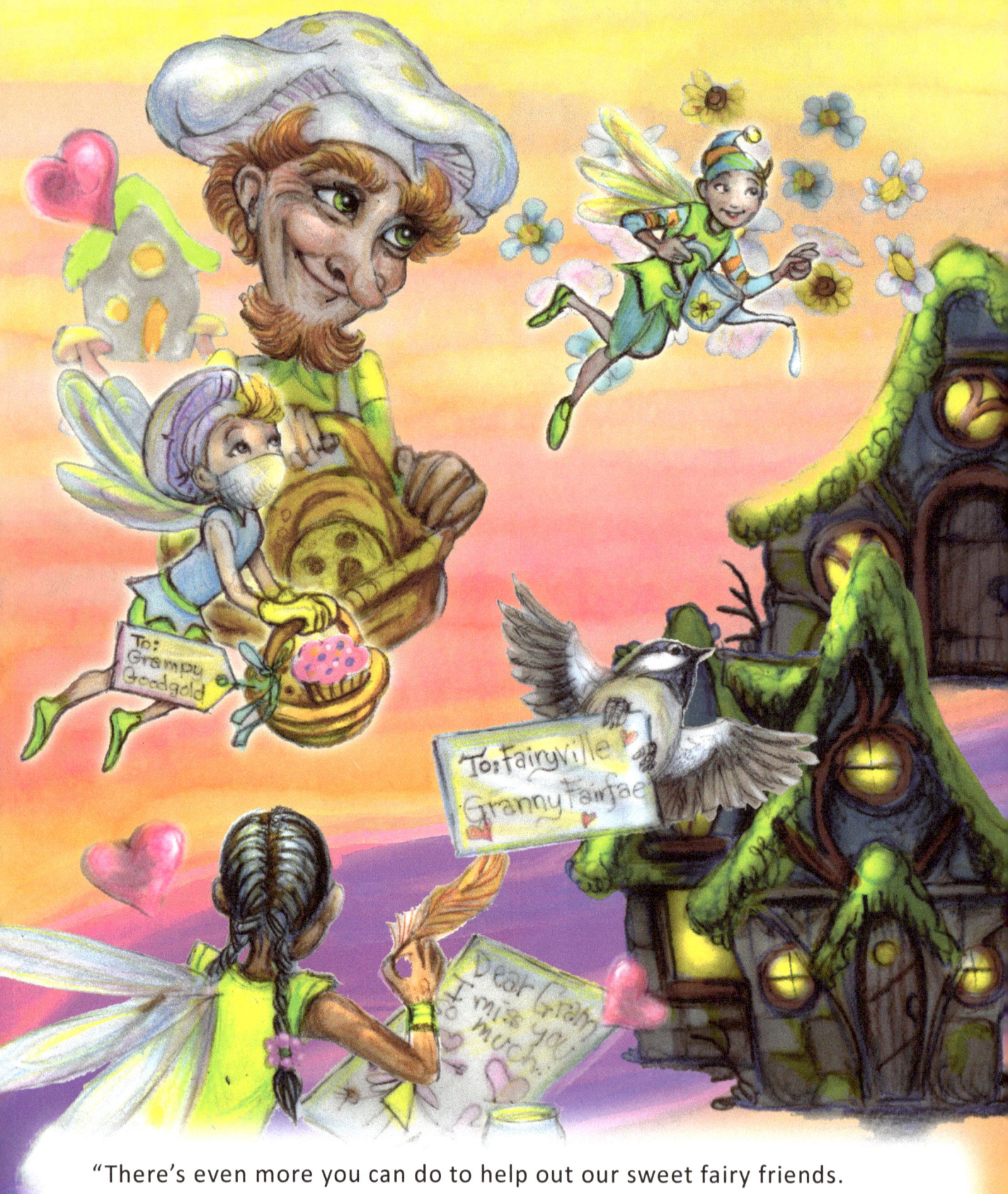

"There's even more you can do to help out our sweet fairy friends.

Stay home, only shop when you must, but no more travel 'til this ends.

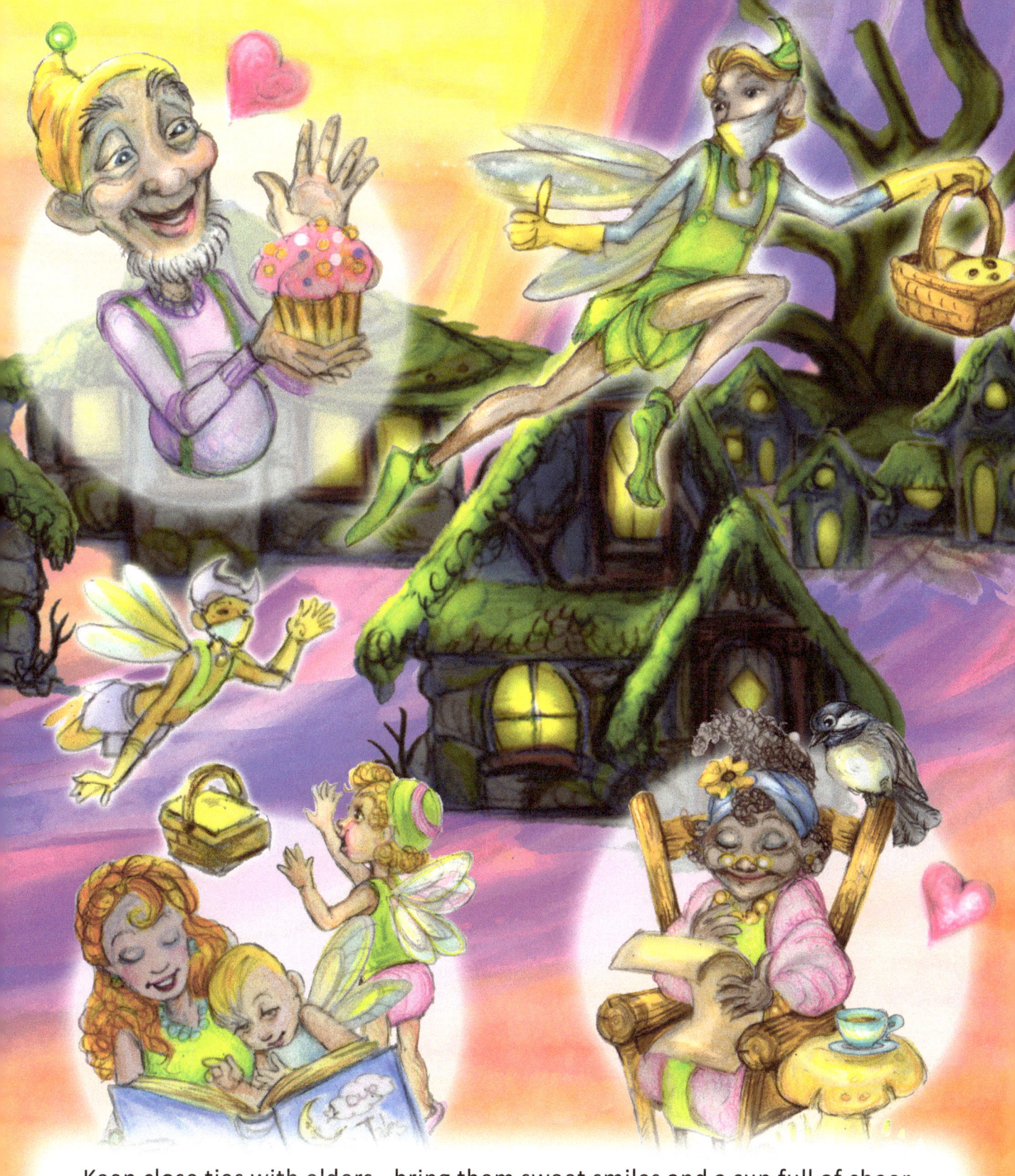

Keep close ties with elders - bring them sweet smiles and a cup full of cheer.

Help out your good Fairyville neighbors, but don't get too close, my dear."

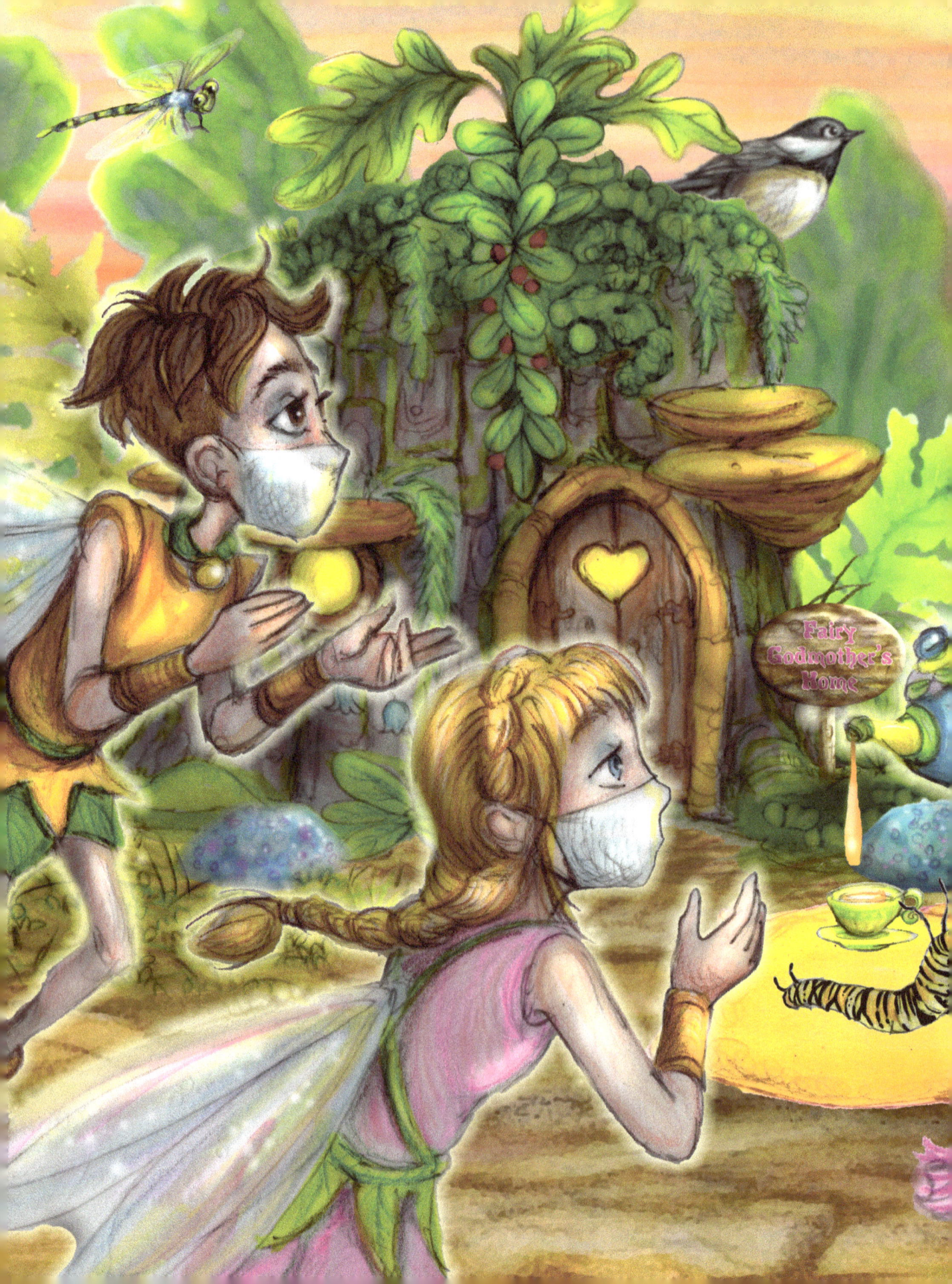

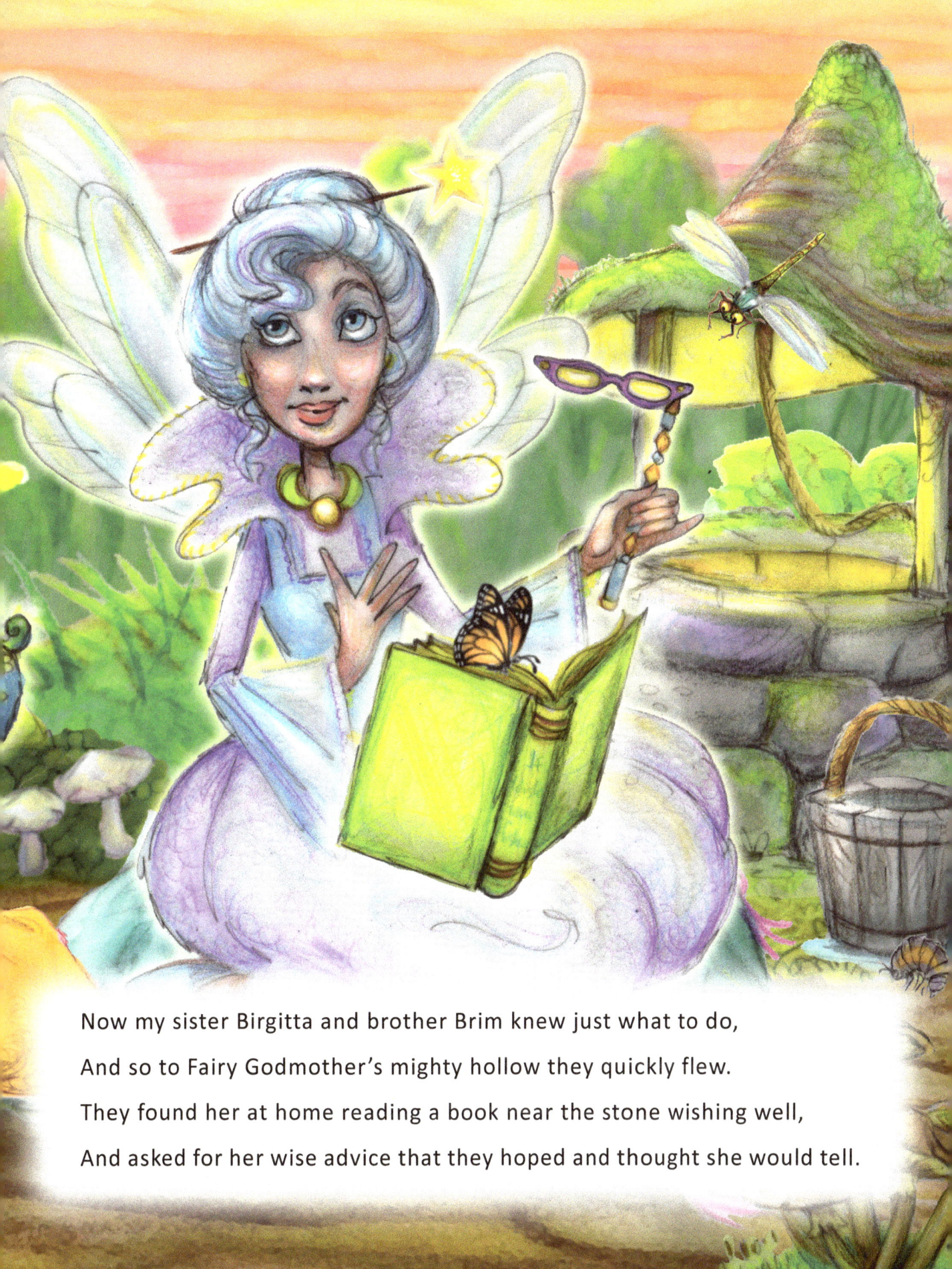

Now my sister Birgitta and brother Brim knew just what to do,

And so to Fairy Godmother's mighty hollow they quickly flew.

They found her at home reading a book near the stone wishing well,

And asked for her wise advice that they hoped and thought she would tell.

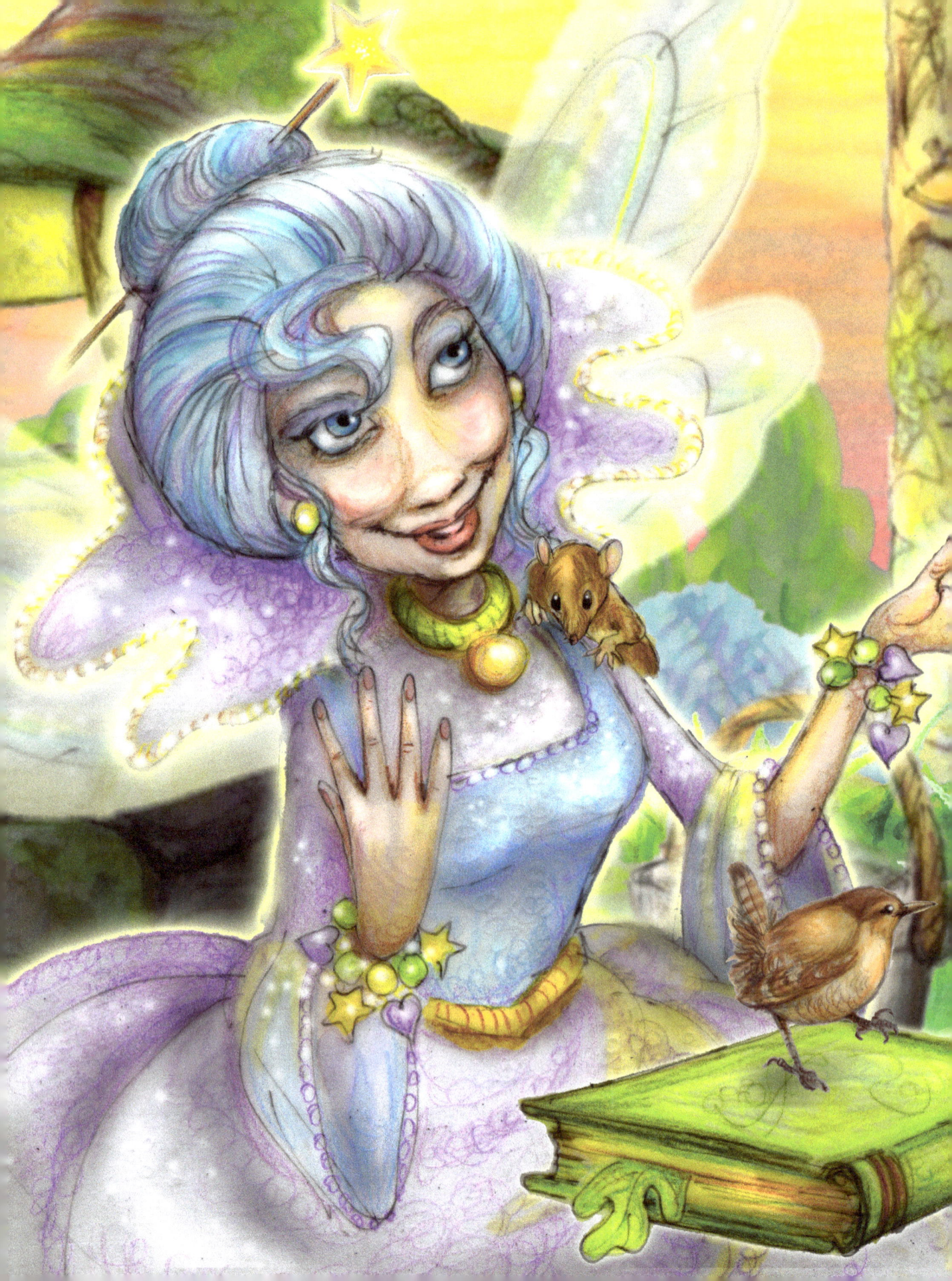

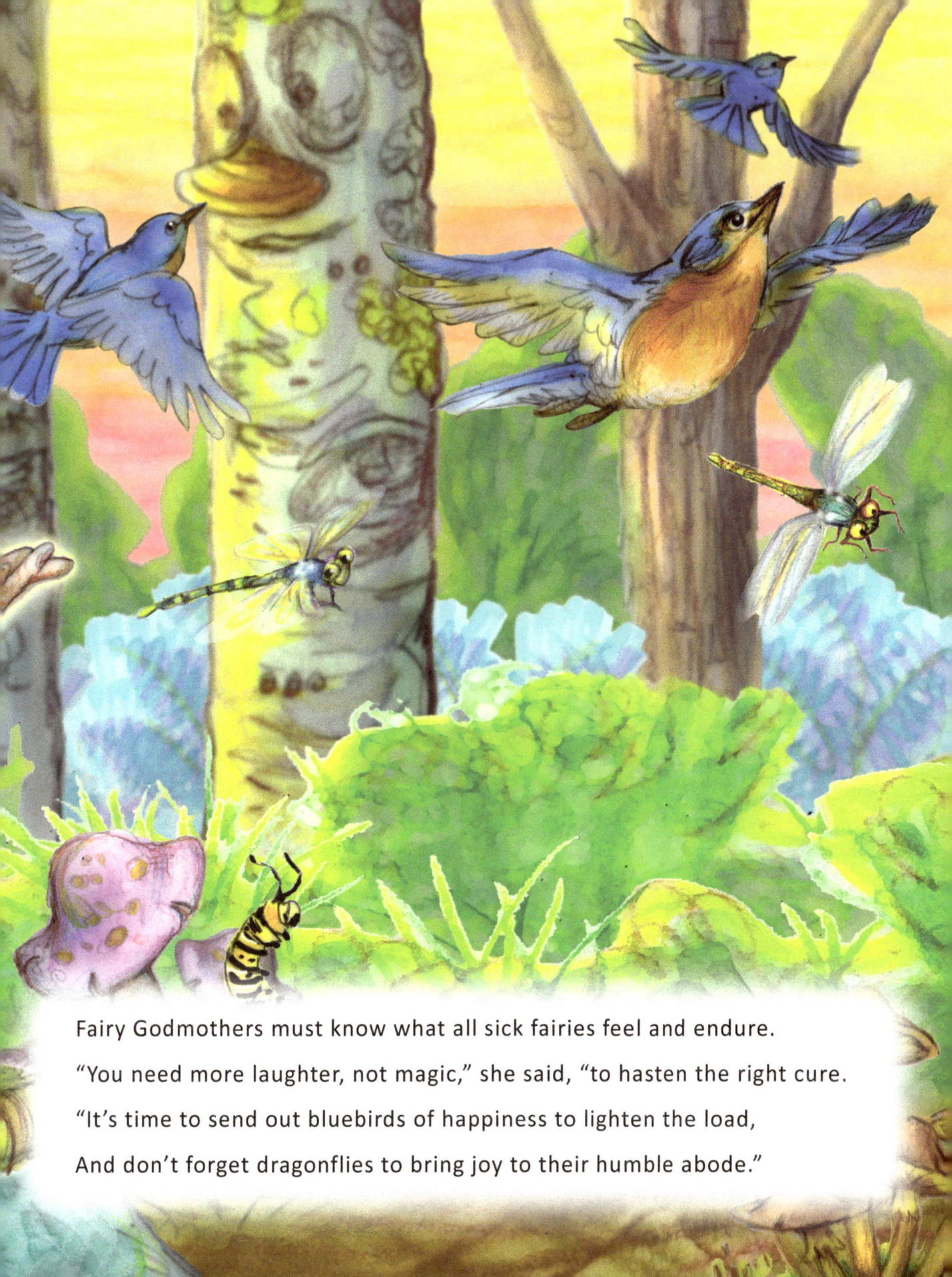

Fairy Godmothers must know what all sick fairies feel and endure.

"You need more laughter, not magic," she said, "to hasten the right cure.

"It's time to send out bluebirds of happiness to lighten the load,

And don't forget dragonflies to bring joy to their humble abode."

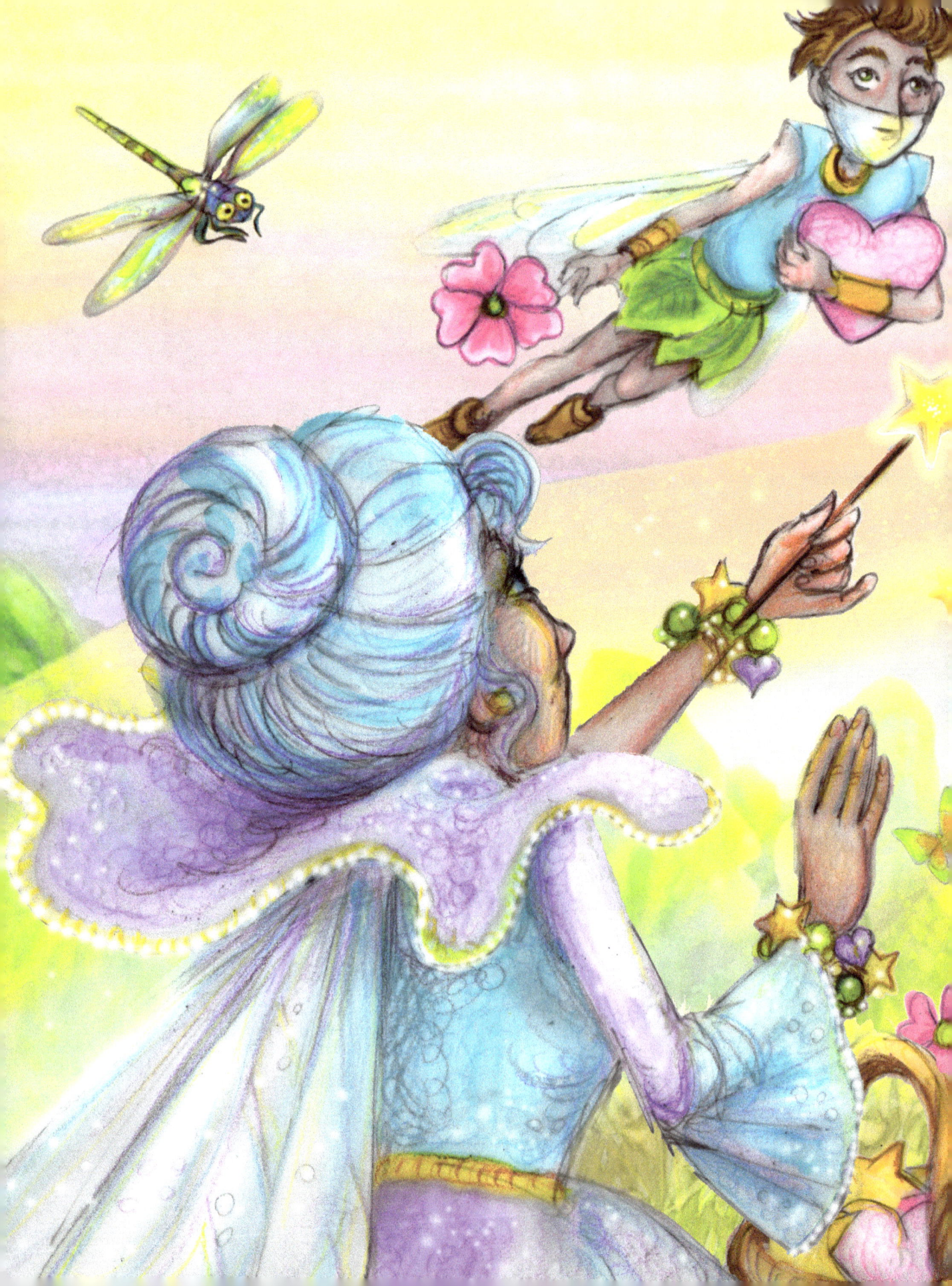

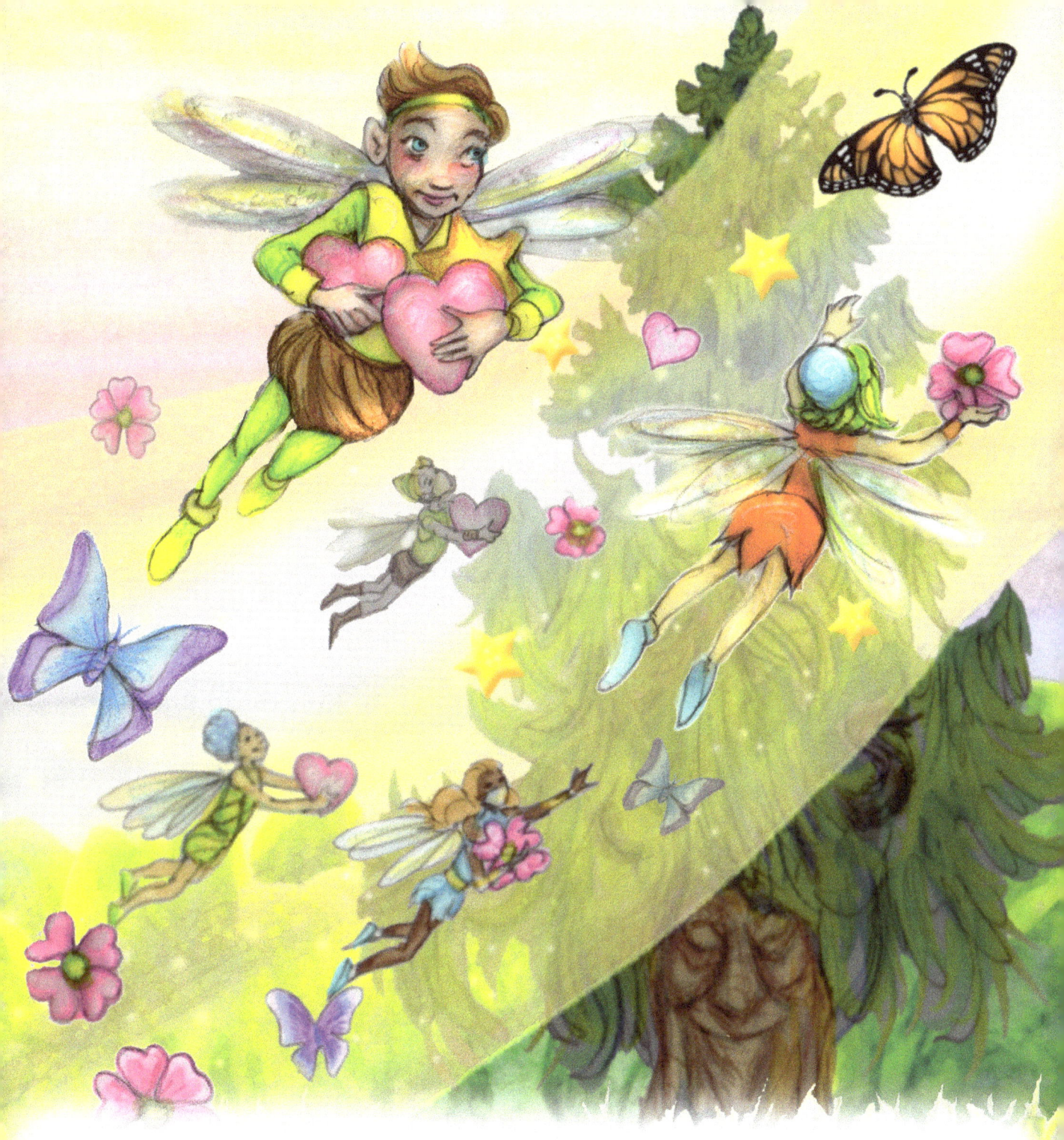

"The hour has come for all fairies to stretch out their smooth, silver wings,

Taking our kindness and hope to other realms and all living things.

Gather your supplies, trooping fairies. You will travel far and near,

Spreading a strong message of love and hope—*they should have no more fear.*"

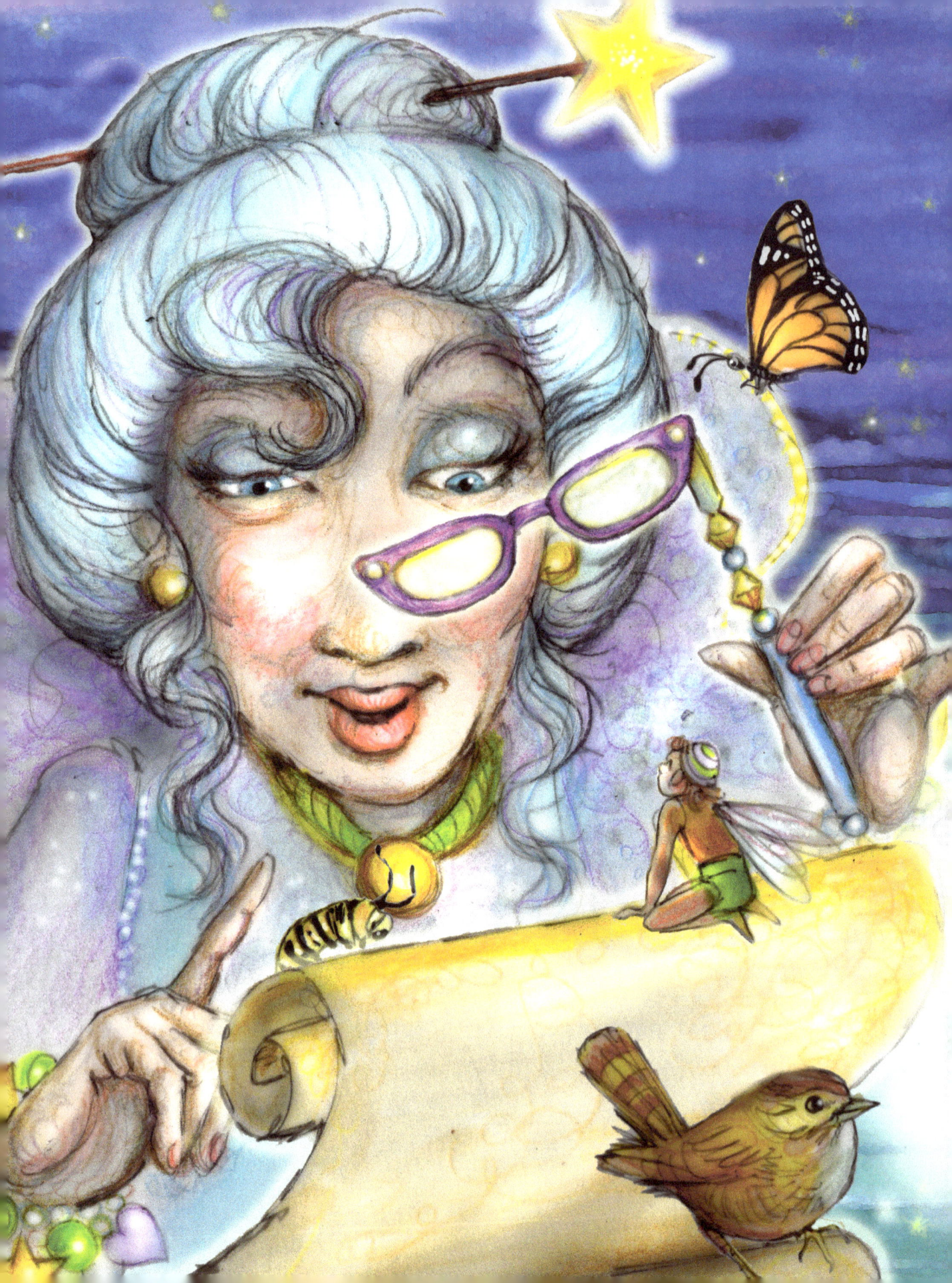

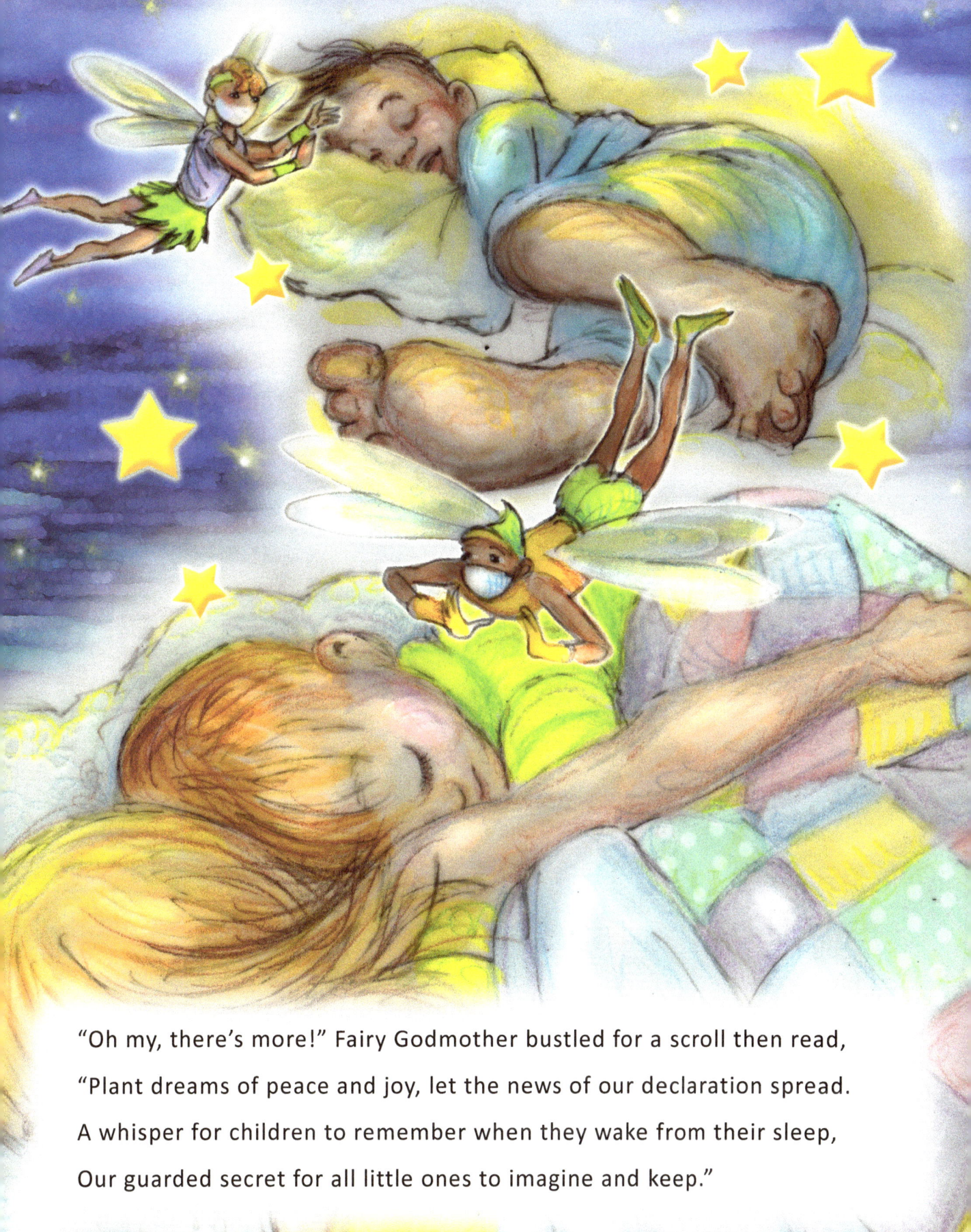

"Oh my, there's more!" Fairy Godmother bustled for a scroll then read,
"Plant dreams of peace and joy, let the news of our declaration spread.
A whisper for children to remember when they wake from their sleep,
Our guarded secret for all little ones to imagine and keep."

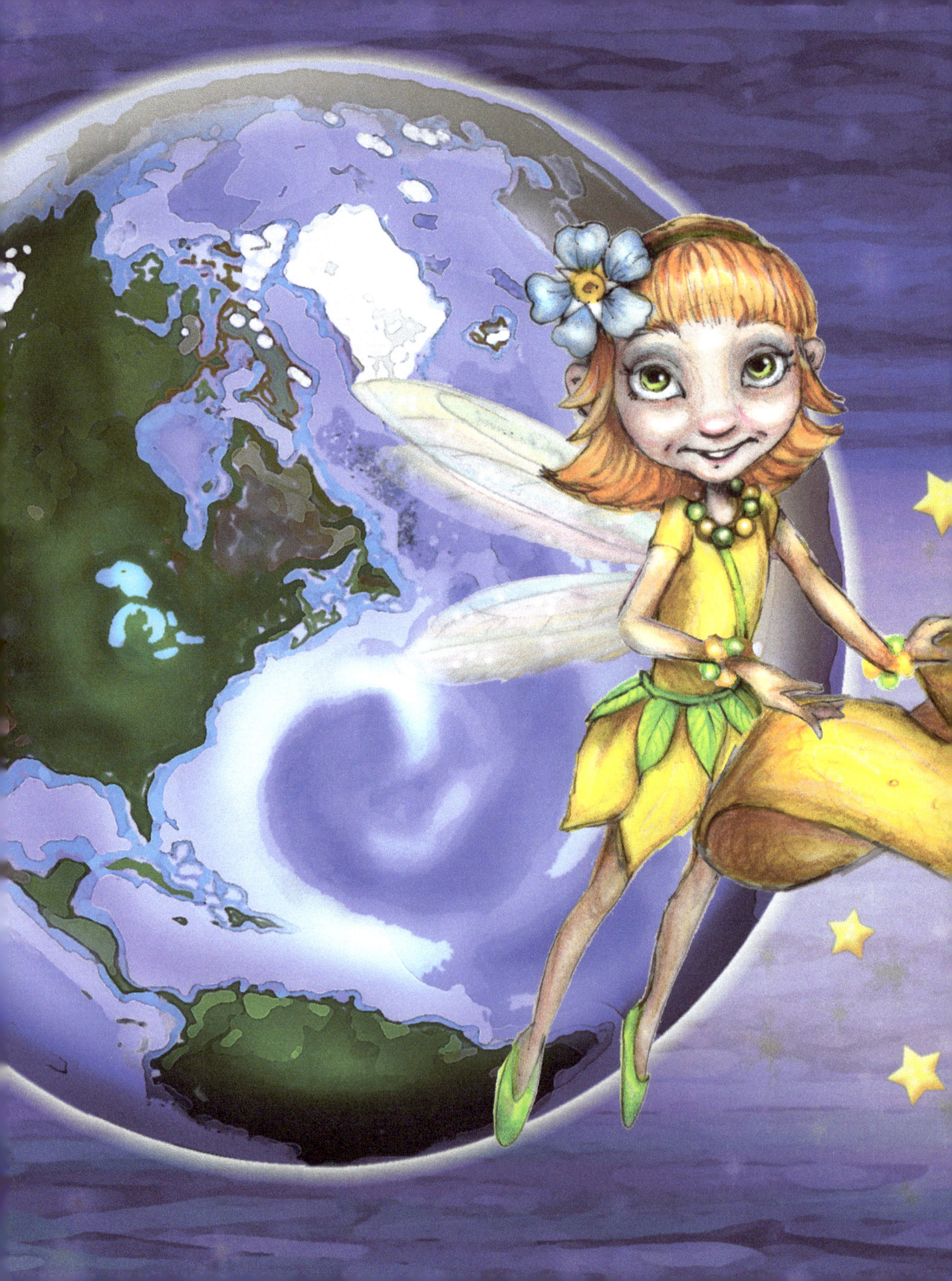

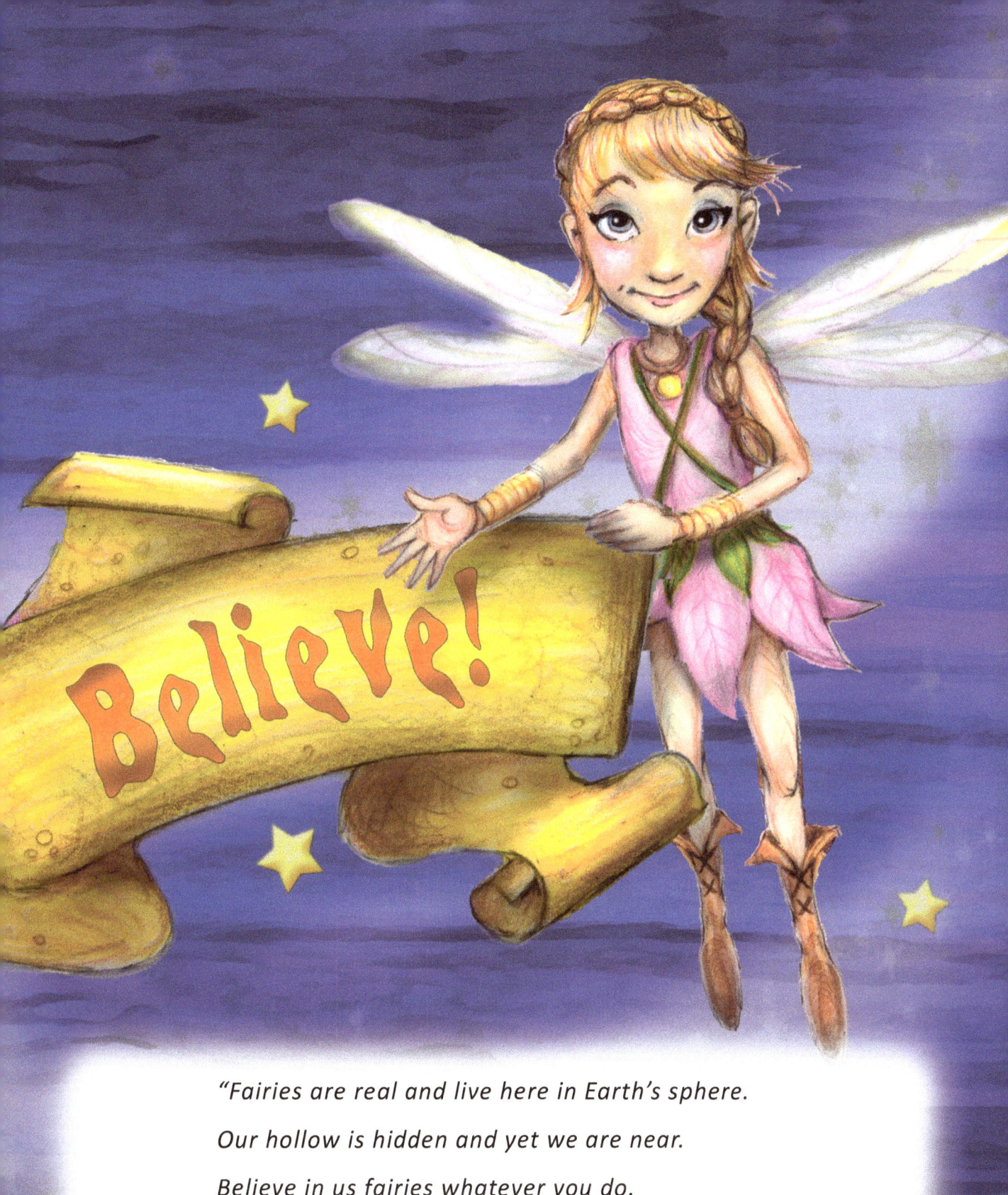

"Fairies are real and live here in Earth's sphere.

Our hollow is hidden and yet we are near.

Believe in us fairies whatever you do.

So our love will shine bright and carry you through."

Join me in the famous words of Peter Pan and declare:

"I Do Believe In Fairies... I Do, I Do, I Do!"

These words brought Tinkerbell back to life, and they can give more energy to fairies everywhere.

Fairy Lore...

1. You can spell fairy in many ways.

If you look in the dictionary, you can see the traditional spelling "fairy". But authors and poets have spelled it, "faerie", "faery", or "fae". The word for fairy is a lot like the fairy beings themselves; they are ever-changing and are not fond about following the rules. Fairies have also been referred to as the gentry, the good people, the fair folk, the little folk, the wee folk, the hill people, and the good neighbors.

2. What is a fairy?

Fairies have been our companions in stories such as, "Cinderella", "Sleeping Beauty", "Pinocchio", and "Peter Pan", but the history of fairies goes way back. The records of fairies can be found in Greek and Roman mythology. But, most of what we know about fairies comes from Celtic mythology. Fairies are nature's guardians of the environment especially trees, flowers, water, and animals.

3. What do legends say about fairies?

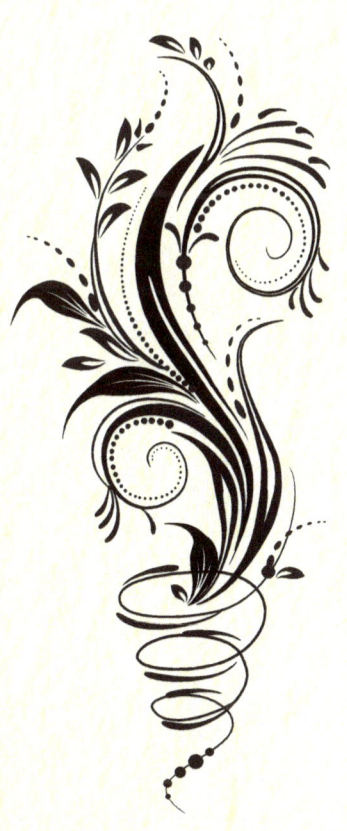

Legends say that the fairies came from Greece and settled in Ireland. They were the Tuatha de' Danaan (pronounced "Thoo-a day Du-non) the descendants of the goddess Danu. It is said, they were a magical race that arrived in Ireland and fought it Celtic inhabitants—known as the Milesians. The Tuatha de' Danaan wanted control over the entire island of Ireland. They created a thick fog that covered the country for three days. During that time, they took control of the land.

However, the Milesians refused to accept this condition and fought back. They wrestled command of the island back from Tuatha de' Danaan, but they could not evict the immortal race. In time, they made an agreement—a *sacred contract with the fairies*. Cleverly, the Milesians allotted themselves the portion of land above the ground and The Tuatha de' Danaan would live in the portion underground—in the hollows and mounds. But, these same *trooping fairies*, as they are known today in Ireland, "continue to *make mischief of one kind or another*".

The powerful trooping fairies of Ireland have always been considered the handsomest of all the fairy kingdom and are considered the aristocracy of the fairy realm. They possess great magic and are skilled in all areas of life. They have the ability to make humans see what they want them to see, or even to see nothing when the fairies wish to remain invisible. Eri, the queen of the Tuatha de' Danaan, requested the island nation be given her name, which they did—Ireland.

4. Where are fairies found?

Fairies live in woodlands and fields and in the hollows of trees. However, when humans began to extend their boundaries, and the forests were claimed and cleared, the fairies began to withdraw. The fairies moved from the great forests to the farms of humans. When fairies and elves continued to lose much of their lands in the Old World, they immigrated to America with the humans, where there was plenty of wilderness. Today fairies and elves live in every country of the world—where nature is freest and wildest.

5. What are the names of fairies in other parts of the world?

Many countries have their own names for nature beings. They were called *elves* in Scandinavia and *trooping fairies* in Britain and Ireland. In Scotland they were called the *seelies* and in Russia they were named the *leshiye*. There were divisions between divisions, but throughout the old world, belief was strong - especially among the Celtic Druids and the Scandinavians.

6. Fairies love gifts and sparkly things.

Fairies love to give gifts and receive them. Their favorite gifts are small shiny objects. It doesn't matter what the object is; they love anything that sparkles or shines. All but the oldest of fairies are easily distracted by a shiny object.

7. Fairies don't like...

Fairies are "allergic" to the metal iron. It makes them feel icky. A fairy can't escape an iron cage, it cancels their magic. Fairies make their own music and shiny bells make them happy, but they carefully avoid bells made by humans which have steel in them (a by-product of iron). Fairies don't like clutter. They dislike those who disrespect or pollute nature. Toxic areas affect fairy health. It is said that fairies do not tell lies and they dislike those that betray secrets.

8. What do fairies do for fun?

Fairies love warm weather, however their favorite holiday is Christmas. They love the Christmas season because of the decorations. They especially love the tinsel on Christmas trees. Fairies rule the winter season and maybe it is because the ice and snow are shiny and sparkly. Fairies usually sleep during the day and come out at night. This makes winter the perfect season for them with its longer time of darkness. Fairies don't like to be seen by people. They can appear and disappear in the blink of an eye. You may never know if you've seen one or not!

9. What do Fairies Do?

Fairies are nature spirits who love the earth. They are guardians of Mother Earth and they want us to be co-guardians of the planet too. Fairies work to help us connect with the earth. Creativity is a magnet for fairies and they assist us in awakening our sense of joy and creativity. They love music, dancing, games, and are known for their musical abilities. Laughter is always an open invitation for them to visit. If stories are being told, fairies gather to listen.

10. Fairy wings.

The wings of a fairy have been described as being similar to a dragonfly or butterfly. They use their wings to wave "hello" to each other. They also make a comfortable cushion when they lie down for a fairy nap.

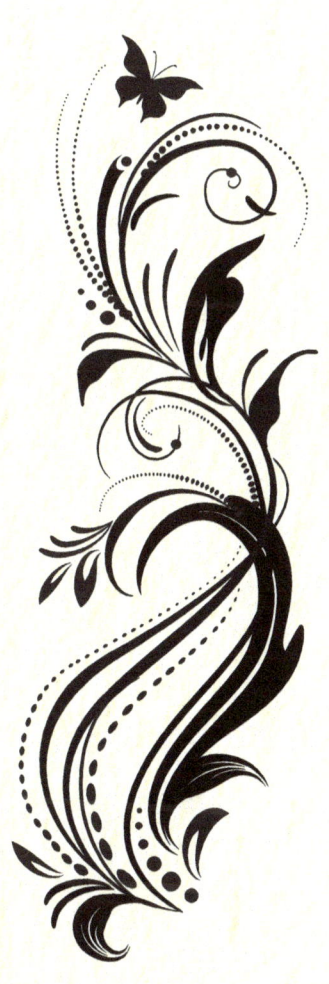

11. Fairy Size.

Fairies are shy creatures. They do not all look the same, but are unique in their own way. Fairies are range in size from the smallest of the flower fairies to the mountain and forest devas. They also have a very pale almost transparent bodies that are in incredibly light. There are male and female fairies.

12. Fairy Abilities.

Like most magical creatures, fairies have special abilities. They have wings which make them able to fly, and they fly quite fast. Fairies are so small and light that they can land on raindrops or dew drops. They can help with one's creativity and imagination. The fairy realm reminds us to keep joy and creativity alive and keep our connection to nature.

13. The best times for fairy encounters...

Look for fairies at the "tween-times" which are the times of dawn, dusk, noon, and midnight. Other important times are the solstices and equinoxes--especially autumn and spring. The fairies are very busy at the spring equinox, (March 21st in the Northern Hemisphere) looking after all the flowers that are blooming. As nature spirits, fairies are drawn to people who do their best to care for Mother Earth. Whistling is a way of calling up the wind which can draw the fairies to you.

14. Fairy Life-Span.

Some say that fairies lived to be 1000 years old. As they age, they slowly lose their glow until they eventually fade away. In the story of Peter Pan by James Matthew Barrie, it is believed that every time someone says "I don't believe in fairies", one of them passes away.

15. What is Troop Night?

"Troop Night" is the fairy version of New Year's Eve. This night with humans is called Halloween. The fairies spend hours from midnight to dawn granting favors and doing good deeds.

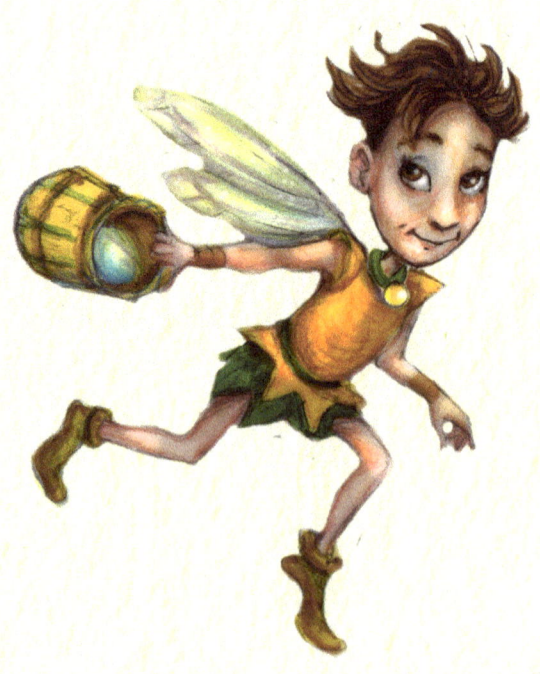

So what are you waiting for?

Lace up your walking boots, get out to the woods and get close to the fairies? However, the fairies may be hard to find, but there is one place where fairyland can always be found, and that is within your own heart.

Resources

Andrew, Ted. *Enchantment of the Faerie Realm*. Woodbury, Minnesota: Llewellyn Publications, 2013.

Curran, Bob. *Irish Fairies*. Belfast, Ireland: Appletree Press Ltd., 2007.

Coughlan, Ronan. *Irish Myths and Legends*. Belfast, Ireland: Appletree Press Ltd., 2007.

Kane, Barry and Tracy. *Fairy Houses Everywhere*. Hong Kong: Paramount Printing Co., 2006.

Moorey, Teresa. *The Fairy Bible*. New York: Sterling Publishing Co., 2008.

Virtue, Doreen. *Fairies 101*. New York: Hay House Ltd., 2013.

For Environmental Resources Go To:

www.caroltrembath.com/resources

About the Author — Carol Trembath

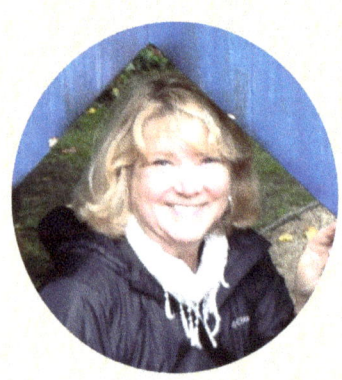

Carol is an award-winning author, Amazon bestseller, and educator of over thirty years. She was awarded a Masters in Library and Information Science from Wayne State University and a Masters in Educational Technology from Michigan State University. Carol is the author of the "Water Walkers Series" which earned the Eric Hoffer "Eye of daVinci" Award for its artwork. The series also won at the Traverse City Moonbeam Awards, a silver and bronze medals in the categories of "Best in Series" and "Multicultural". In 2019 Carol's latest publication, "Out of Slavery: A Novel of Harriet Tubman", won a silver medal at the same awards in the category of "Best First Novel". www.caroltrembath.com

About the Illustrator — Lori Taylor

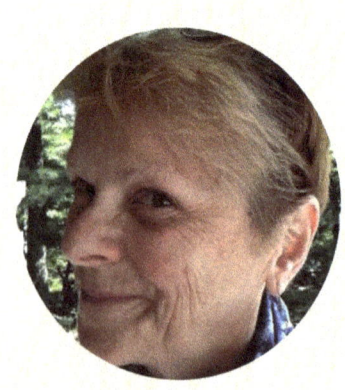

Lori Taylor is a Michigan artist/author/illustrator. She is a freelance illustrator who has created many children's educational exhibits for Michigan nature centers, and selected as artist-in-residence for the Sleeping Bear Dunes National Lakeshore, the Porcupine Mountains Wilderness State Park, and the Literacy Legacy Fund of Michigan. Her books were selected as a "Great Lakes, Great Reads" from the Historical Society of Michigan and her illustrations have won awards at Michigan art fairs. www.loritaylorart.com

www.ingramcontent.com/pod-product-compliance
Lightning Source LLC
Chambersburg PA
CBHW041200100726
47911CB00016B/810